LIZ EARLE'S
QUICK GUIDES

Food
Combining

LIZ EARLE'S
QUICK GUIDES

Food Combining

B❋XTREE

Advice to the Reader

Before following any dietary advice contained in this book, it is
recommended that you consult your doctor if you suffer from any health
problems or special condition or are in any doubt.

First published in Great Britain in 1995 by Boxtree Limited,
Broadwall House, 21 Broadwall, London SE1 9PL

10 9 8 7 6 5 4 3 2 1

ISBN: 0 7522 1673 2

Text design by Blackjacks
Cover design by Hammond Hammond

Printed and Bound in Great Britain by Cox & Wyman Ltd.,
Reading, Berkshire

A CIP catalogue entry for this book is available from
the British Library

Contents

Introduction

The concept of food combining for health and weight-loss was developed by Dr Hay seventy odd years ago. His original concept of 'don't mix the foods that fight' has since been followed by literally millions of devotees around the world. By this, Dr Hay meant separating the foods that are difficult to digest together. This gives the body the opportunity to use food more efficiently and helps to prevent our insides becoming clogged and sluggish. Although the scientific support for this system is slight, there is overwhelming anecdotal evidence that this way of eating increases energy levels and aids weight-loss. I have personally spoken to many hundreds of people who have benefited from the simple rule of not mixing starch with protein. The principles of food combining really are very straightforward and this *Quick Guide* gives all you need to know in order to improve your own health and well-being.

Liz Earle

ACKNOWLEDGEMENTS

I am grateful to Sarah Hamilton Fleming for helping to produce this book. Also to Dr Ann Walker, Lecturer in human nutrition at the University of Reading for her technical expertise. I am also indebted to the talented team at Boxtree, and to Rosemary Sandberg and Claire Bowles Publicity for their unfailing enthusiasm and support.

1

The History of Food Combining

Food, glorious food, is essential for life. Once absorbed by our bodies it provides us with energy and the nutrients we need to form strong, healthy cells. All we see of the food we eat is what comes out the other end, and most of us have very little idea of what happens to it in between. Even today, medics do not know *exactly* what is involved in digesting food and it remains one of the secrets of life. However, we do know that food is both life giving and life destroying and one man's meal is another man's poison. As an example, eating a single peanut can be life threatening to someone with a severe allergy to peanuts, although it is perfectly harmless to others. It is, therefore, important that we eat the right kinds of food. Even those who do not have a serious digestive illness, such as a food allergy or inflammatory bowel disease, may suffer from minor digestive disorders, like indigestion and flatulence, as a result of eating the wrong combinations of food. This *Quick Guide* is all about a system of eating which is designed to improve our digestive processes by making sure that we do not mix the foods that fight!

It is only very recently that the medical profession has become aware of the importance of nutrition and begun to acknowledge that we are what we eat. Doctors have always known that we need food to survive, but in the past they paid little attention to how essential some foods are and how damaging others can be. Now it is known that a huge variety of disorders and ailments, mental and physical (some of which are very severe), are caused by a diet lacking in vital nutrients, and these conditions can often be cured by simply changing what we eat. Eating healthily is something we can all do to keep our bodies in good working order and minimise the risk of illness. Unfortunately, conventional doctors are only just beginning to recognise the importance of diet and many are reluctant to suggest dietary changes to their patients.

Being overweight is another sign that the body is unhealthy. Many people simply accept being overweight as their unfortunate lot in life and that there is little they can do about it. This is untrue. Our bodies can carry out numerous complex processes simultaneously. Imagine trying to cook a meal, watch television, write a letter and talk to someone on the telephone all at the same time. You couldn't – it would be impossible, but your body can; every day, like some vast computer, and its ability to maintain a comfortable and healthy weight is just one of the many processes of self-preservation. If we fight against these natural body processes by eating large amounts of fattening, processed foods, the body will become overloaded and will have trouble in assimilating and then eliminating them. As a result, the food is stored in the body as fat and toxins, which can build up and contribute to heart disease and other degenerative illnesses. Too many people still think of fat in a purely cosmetic light as something which is merely unattractive. But being heavily overweight is a sign of ill-health. Believe it or not, food combining can help us to lose weight permanently while cleansing our bodies and generally boosting our all-round health.

Diet and Degenerative Disease

This subject could easily take up the entire book, as there has been so much research carried out into the importance of diet in disease prevention. Today, almost everyone knows that fruit and vegetables are good for us and millions of pounds have been invested in researching exactly which nutrients present in these foods are so beneficial. It is now known that the antioxidant effects of the vitamins A (in the form of beta-carotene), C and E play a major role in the fight against free radicals. It is thought that an excess of free radicals is largely responsible for the cell damage involved in cancer, heart disease, all degenerative diseases and even the ageing process itself. But fruit and vegetables don't just contain a handful of vitamins. They are also a rich source of water, fibre and enzymes, which aid our digestive and elimination processes. Considering that human beings are 70 percent water, it is important that our water levels are continuously replenished and the most effective way of achieving this is by eating foods with a high water content, such as fruit and vegetables.

Food combining allows us to make the best of our food. It encourages us to eat as much fresh fruit and vegetables as possible and never to mix starch with protein as this interferes with our digestive processes. Food combining is a very simple concept based on eating healthy natural foods that the body can utilise effectively. As long as you do not mix 'the foods that fight', you can eat as many of the 'right' foods as you like and, instead of putting on weight, you will actually lose it. Your energy levels should soar and a whole range of seemingly incurable ailments, such as headaches and even depression, may improve or even disappear entirely. If you do not believe that eating the right food can have such a dramatic effect on your general health and weight, then try talking to someone who suffers from a food allergy or food intolerance. For these people, giving up the irritating food, be it wheat or nuts, can cure headaches, severe depression and violent skin rashes. Many people have experienced the same results with food combining. Food is our fuel and without it we will die, but eating the wrong foods can be just as damaging, in the same way that filling a car with the wrong kind of petrol will make the engine unable to function properly.

Food combining is an easy eating plan designed for life and not merely a temporary diet. If you try food combining for a couple of weeks, you should notice a dramatic increase in your energy levels, weight-loss and healthy skin. You will probably wish to continue to reap these benefits from food combining. Not many diets allow you to eat as much food as you like but food combining does! So whether you take up food combining to lose weight or simply to detox your body and boost your energy levels, you will never have to deprive yourself of food. At first sight food combining may seem somewhat complicated, but once you have understood the theory behind it you will see that it is a diet based firmly on common sense. However, be warned – you will have to give up many traditional meals, such as meat and potatoes, pizza, lasagne and most sandwiches. This will be difficult at first, but it is easy to adapt recipes so that carbohydrates and proteins are not combined. Neither is there any need for your meals to lack variety.

The Pioneer of Food Combining

The concept of food combining for health originated in America during the latter part of the nineteenth century. For the first sixteen years of his career, Dr Howard Hay had practised conventional medicine until he became very ill at the age of forty with Bright's disease (a serious kidney condition). He had high blood pressure and a dilated heart and, as conventional medicine offered no cure, he decided to seek his own. He did this through food alone and, after three months on a diet consisting mostly of raw food, Dr Hay's symptoms gradually disappeared and he felt fitter than he had done for years. This confirmed his growing suspicion that medicine was on the wrong track in attempting to treat the symptoms of disease instead of the cause.

Dr Hay firmly believed 'that the body is merely a composite of what goes into it daily in the form of food and drink.' It was this conviction that prompted him to develop the system for eating which made him famous – the Hay system of food combining. He claimed that eating the right foods at the right time enabled the body to remain strong and healthy. Food combining works on the principle that certain foods should not be eaten together, namely proteins and starches, because mixing these foods inhibits their digestion. Dr Hay thought that *all* diseases are caused by the wrong chemical conditions in the body. Eating the wrong mixtures of foods leads to an over-accumulation of acids (the natural end-products of digestion and metabolism) and that this is responsible for the wrong chemical conditions. As the body is unable to eliminate these acids they decay inside the body, poisoning it.

To avoid this build-up of toxic acids within the body, Dr Hay advised his patients to avoid eating much meat and too many refined carbohydrates (eg sugar and products made from white flour). According to his theory, we build up a tolerance to eating these 'bad' foods and this reduces our vitality. He found that, once someone adopts his system of eating and does not mix starches with proteins, if they return to their previous eating habits their stomach will immediately react to the 'bad' food.

Although this makes sense to the majority of us today, Dr Hay's theories were frowned upon and ridiculed by the medical profession at the time and he received a barrage of criticism. It is not difficult to imagine doctors thinking of Dr Hay as a quack, considering the ignorance of some medics today when it comes to diet and nutrition. Despite the fact that Dr Hay cured many patients of supposedly incurable ailments through his food-combining diet, this did not hold any water with his professional colleagues. However, he did find some acceptance from doctors who attended his lectures. Ironically, it was not until after Dr Hay died in 1940 that the medical profession as a whole began to investigate the link between nutrition and health.

Today, medical authorities are shifting their approach by investigating methods of disease prevention and dealing with the causes of disease rather then just the symptoms. Governments around the world are investing millions of pounds in nutritional research to come up with a cheap and effective way of preventing many diseases, including cancer and heart disease (our biggest killers – heart disease causes 40 percent of deaths each year!). Medical authorities are excited by the potential of preventing illness through diet as it is not only cheaper than using drugs, it is also perfectly safe, unlike many conventional drug treatments which can have harmful side-effects. The Hay system is not a cure-all, but one of the healthiest ways of eating and it not only advises which foods we need the most, but it also takes into consideration how our bodies make the best use of these foods.

How Food Combining Works

The most important rule to remember when food combining is not to mix carbohydrates with proteins and acid fruits. **Proteins** refer to concentrated animal proteins (20 percent or more) such as meat, poultry, fish and cheese. **Carbohydrates** are concentrated starches (20 percent or more), such as grains, bread and cereals and potatoes. Sugars also fall into this category.

Following this fundamental principle of food combining, here are five basic rules of thumb:

* Starches and sugars should not be eaten with proteins and acid fruits at the same meal

* The diet should consist mainly of vegetables, salads and fruits
* All processed and refined foods should be avoided and ideally only wholegrain carbohydrates should be eaten, such as wholemeal bread, pasta and brown rice. White flour, sugar and processed fats, in particular, should be avoided
* Proteins, starches and fats should be eaten in moderation only
* There should be at least a four-hour interval between meals of different character.

Starch and Protein Digestion

Dr Hay had good reason for advising his patients not to combine starch and protein in the same meal, because they can conflict during the process of digestion. When animal proteins reach the stomach, the body releases hydrochloric acid, which activates the enzyme known as pepsin. This enzyme has the important job of splitting the proteins and absorbing them and the process can only take place in a completely acid environment. Eating carbohydrates upsets the acid medium and this interferes with the digestion of proteins. Followers of the Hay system believe the undigested protein can have a serious impact on our health, because the body is unable to utilise it and may have trouble removing this leftover waste effectively.

Dr Hay believed that the half-digested protein rots inside the body and is stored inside us. The body attempts to keep this toxic waste well away from our vital organs and so it often stores it in fatty deposits in the skin, known as cellulite. However, if there is a significant build-up of toxins they will eventually affect our internal organs and contribute to the development of disease.

Similarly, the body requires an alkaline medium in order to digest carbohydrates. Digestion is initiated in the mouth by the action of the enzyme ptyalin, which splits the starches before they enter the small intestine, where they are digested further. (It is important that all foods are thoroughly chewed otherwise the small intestine will be unable to digest the food properly.) In the stomach, saliva containing the active ptyalin is mixed with the starches. This digestive phase lasts for approximately thirty to forty-five minutes. However, if meat, or other acid-forming foods, are added to this alkaline mixture, the splitting-down process of starches is stopped and these half-digested foods ferment in the stomach.

There have been a number of small scientific studies to support this theory. One early study carried out by three Philadelphia investigators in 1936 on five subjects revealed the amount of acidity in the stomach after protein meals, after starch meals, and after combined starch and protein meals. The results showed that, at one and a quarter hours after these meals were eaten, the stomach contents after the high protein meal were mostly acid; they were least acid after a high starch meal and they were halfway between the two states after a mixed meal. More significantly, the stomach contents after the combined meal revealed that the proteins were not being digested properly as the acid level was far lower than that which is required for an all-protein meal. The level of acidity had actually been reduced by two-thirds due to the presence of the starch foods. To put it simply, when starch and protein are eaten together, the alkaline components of the starch interfere with the digestion of the protein, and the acidity accompanying the protein foods likewise hinders the digestion of the starches.

This contrasts with the conventional theory that, when eating any kind of food, we produce gastric juice containing hydrochloric acid, and this destroys the alkaline medium. However, the protein present in carbohydrates, such as grains, is very small (about 10 percent) and is incomplete. Therefore, starches do not stimulate enough hydrochloric acid to interfere with the alkaline medium that is required for their digestion.

Nevertheless, many doctors today disagree with Dr Hay's explanation of the starch–protein theory and maintain that the gastric juice is necessary for the splitting of the starches. The starch is often contained in what are known as 'protein envelopes' which require the acid action so that the starch can be released from these envelopes. This is correct, but it does not alter the fact that the initial stage of starch digestion occurs in an alkaline medium for the first thirty minutes or so that it is in the stomach. After that, there is plenty of time for the gastric acid to digest the starches before they enter the small intestine. There, the pancreatic juice completes the digestion of carbohydrates and protein in a mostly alkaline medium. In the end, whichever theory is true does not really matter to the thousands of people in Britain alone who have found that food combining works.

2

Food Combining for Health

Nature's Diet

On first inspection, food combining may appear to be a frighteningly complicated eating regime in which the majority of traditional meals are banned. However, it is far more natural to eat in the way that food combining dictates than to eat meals that contain all major food groups. Anthropological and archaeological evidence shows that our ancestors, the hunter-gatherers, had a healthy existence on a high-alkaline diet of berries, shoots, nuts and seeds (the gathered food) with occasional meat (the hunted food). The gathered food would have been eaten in its natural state and, although the meat would have been cooked, it would not have been served up with potatoes and cabbage or tossed in some spaghetti! The stone-age diet was rich in fibre and fresh produce whereas today we clog our bodies with a combination of processed carbohydrates and proteins which are often high in sugar and saturated fat. Our digestive system has trouble assimilating the resulting mess that ends up in the stomach. It is only comparatively recently that we have combined the different food groups and included processed food in our diet. Today, we also eat far too many refined carbohydrates in the form of sugar, white bread, pasta and rice, too many of the wrong kinds of fat and not enough fibre and fresh produce. Food combining brings us closer to the natural diet of our forebears who, by all accounts, were far healthier and suffered far less from obesity and degenerative diseases than we do today.

Keeping in Chemical Balance

As we have seen, the chemical balance of our digestive system determines how well we digest our food and this ultimately has an effect on our health and even whether we store food as fat! For optimum health, our diet should consist of four times as much alkali-forming foods as acid-forming foods. According to one of Dr Hay's influential advocate, Doris Grant, when he was asked about the scientific basis for the ratio, he replied:

> We have no way of arriving at the relative proportion of alkaline and acid elements needed by the body except through an analysis of its excretions. When we take into account all of the excretions through the four avenues of elimination, we find that the loss in alkali is four times as great as that in acid. This means that if we would replace our losses fully we need four times as much of the alkaline intake as of the acid intake. This is a fact well known to physiologists and can be verified in almost any work on physiology.

The End-products of Food

After all the food we eat is digested, the end-product is either acidic or alkaline. What we eat determines this chemical balance. It must be stressed here that, although both concentrated starches and concentrated proteins are 'acid-forming', this has no bearing on the fact that starches need an alkaline medium and proteins need an acid medium for their digestion.

If we eat too many acid-forming foods, ie concentrated carbohydrates and proteins, then the end-products will be highly acidic, and this can cause a number of unpleasant symptoms, such as gas, flatulence, heartburn and acid indigestion. Furthermore, if we combine these concentrated foods, the digestion, assimilation and elimination of both types of food is hindered and this can cause a build-up of toxic waste which may affect our health, both in the short term and the long term.

Alkali-forming foods. These include all vegetables except potatoes (unless they are cooked in their skins and the skins are eaten); all fresh fruit (except cranberries and plums); almonds and milk.

Acid-forming foods. These include all animal proteins such as meat, poultry, fish, shellfish, cheese, eggs and nuts (except almonds); all carbohydrates such as grains, bread and flour, pasta and other foods made from cereal starches, and sugars.

For a more extensive list of the different foods in each category, see the table at the end of Chapter 4.

In order to reach the 4:1 alkali–acid ratio, you should have the following meals each day:

* one protein meal
* one starch meal
* one wholly alkaline meal.

To boost your health from time to time, it is a good idea to have the occasional day when you eat nothing but frequent meals of one kind of fruit – a great way to detox. Fresh fruit is very easy to digest, especially when you eat only one variety, as the enzymes present in many fruit and vegetables aid the processes of digestion, assimilation and elimination.

Inner Cleansing and Detoxification

Recent research has revealed that the health of a nation depends upon what its people eat. For example, Mediterraneans have a much lower risk of suffering from heart attacks and strokes than Britons, and this has been linked to a traditional diet containing mostly fresh produce and olive oil. The link between diet and health is now well established, but the food industry continues to promote highly processed, less healthy products, often with evasive or misleading marketing. It is due to modern eating habits that the majority of us will have some build-up of toxins within our bodies, some more than others. Adopting this food-combining plan will stimulate our bodies to release these toxins so that they can at last be eliminated.

Once you have unburdened your system your body will be better equipped to lose weight and fight illness. It is important to bear in mind that these toxins may have built up over a period of many years and so their elimination is not going to occur overnight. During the first week of food combining, you may experience headaches, body aches, bloating, diarrhoea or constipation. This is a result of your body adjusting to a completely new diet and the fact that toxins are being released suddenly from where they are stored within the body in order to be eliminated. You may also experience cold symptoms such as a runny nose, but this is because your body is trying to eliminate toxins which have been stored in the mucous membranes. These symptoms of the detoxification process will pass after a few days and will soon be replaced with renewed energy levels and improved all-round health.

Natural Body Cycles

Every day the food we eat is digested by the body, assimilated and then finally eliminated. Many nutritionists now believe that we carry out each of these processes in natural cycles. It is thought that, from midday to 8pm, we are busy digesting our daily intake of food – this is known as appropriation. Then, through the night from 8pm until 4am, our bodies are actively assimilating the food – that is, absorbing all the nutrients in the digested food and making use of these. Finally, from 4am until midday, our bodies eliminate the remainder of the food which is now waste material. This all makes perfect sense although, unfortunately, we often disrupt these natural cycles by eating at the wrong time – especially late at night. Many find that, after eating large amounts of food late at night, they feel groggy the following morning. This is probably because, instead of our bodies being able to assimilate the food and start the elimination process, they are still busy digesting it. We need to make the best use of these body cycles in order to lose weight and maintain optimum health. Those who eat too much will be spending most of their time appropriating the food, leaving little time for the body to assimilate the nutrients from it and eliminate the waste material. This may be one reason why the food gets stored as fat.

A Cure for Minor Ailments

There are a number of minor ailments which doctors accept are caused or sometimes aggravated by diet. These include indigestion, constipation, obesity, arthritis, allergy, skin diseases, the common cold, headaches and diabetes mellitus. Dr Hay's devotees claim that all of these conditions can be considerably improved or even cured by adopting food combining in the long term.

INDIGESTION
The symptoms of indigestion – abdominal pain, heartburn and flatulence – are common. Indigestion is usually caused by

mixing the wrong foods together, thus causing a build-up of toxic acid in the stomach. When proteins and carbohydrates are combined, the digestion of both is blocked to some extent and both foods may ferment and create toxic acids within the body. When you think about it, it is hardly surprising that fermenting, semi-digested food clogging up thirty feet of intestines often causes discomfort.

This can easily be remedied by ensuring that these foods are no longer combined. Indigestion pains are most commonly caused by cheese sandwiches, or meat and bread mixed together. Instead of changing their diet to eradicate this cause of indigestion, many sufferers try to alleviate the symptoms by taking antacids. Dr Hay warned against this, claiming that these can lead to further trouble. It is thought that some antacids can use up specific vitamins in the body which are essential for certain bodily processes. Dr Ann Walker, lecturer in human nutrition at the University of Reading, explains that many of the ingredients in antacids interfere with other processes. One of the most common antacid ingredients is aluminium hydroxide, which interferes with the absorption of calcium, iron, magnesium and phosphorus. Calcium and phosphorus are needed for healthy bones and the elderly, in particular, need to maintain their levels of these vital nutrients. Sodium bicarbonate is also present in some antacids and this interferes with the absorption of folic acid, so pregnant women should avoid taking antacids. Even the antacids which contain more useful minerals, such as magnesium, are known to have the side-effect of causing diarrhoea. In the short term, people may not notice any problems as a result of taking antacids, but the long-term consequences could be serious. As Dr Walker says, 'What is worrying is that those who take antacids for their indigestion tend to take them regularly and rely on them. It is another case of people treating the symptoms of a condition when they should be dealing with its cause, which may involve stress or be diet related.'

Another common cause of indigestion is eating too quickly and not chewing properly. To get the most from our food, it is best to eat in a relaxed environment where we can sit down and savour every mouthful. Many of us lead such busy lives that we end up grabbing a sandwich and eating on the run. Few people realise how important it is to chew every mouthful thoroughly to enable our body to digest the food properly. When we chew something, we decrease the size of food particles; this increases the food's surface area, making it easier for enzymes to do their job of breaking down the food. This breaking-down process enables our bodies to utilise all the nutrients in the food without building up excessive wastes. Chewing also produces salivary amylase enzymes which digest carbohydrates.

If there is a lot of fat in your diet, this will hinder the digestive process because it inhibits the secretion of gastric acid and the enzyme pepsin in the stomach.

CONSTIPATION

Dr Hay blamed constipation as being one of the main sources of acid formation and he warned that long periods of constipation could contribute to the development of a number of degenerative diseases, including cancer of the colon. Today, many medics acknowledge that constipation is one of the main causes of cancer of the bowel in the developed world. Dr Hay and other scientists believed that a diet comprising too much refined carbohydrate and acid-forming meat and not enough fibre is responsible for constipation. He also believed that combining carbohydrate and protein is at the root of the problem and this was supported in a paper called *Amylaceous Dyspepsia* (starch-caused indigestion), written by Dr Lionel J. Picton in 1938. In this particular paper, Dr Picton highlighted a well-known laboratory experiment on dogs by the famous Russian scientist, Pavlov. Pavlov had discovered that a dog digests minced beef in about four hours and starch in about an hour and a half. However, when meat was mixed with starch there was a considerable delay in digestion and the meal took eight hours or more to leave the stomach. Dr Picton suggested that the delay in digestion indicates delays all along the line: 'The somewhat startling conclusion flows from this, that meals of mixed character such as meat and bread favour constipation, whereas meat and salad at one meal and starchy food such as bread and butter at a separate meal have no such effect.'

This paper also contained case histories of patients who had benefited from food combining. By removing the cause of constipation, ie too much acid-forming meat and refined carbohydrates, from the diet and increasing our intake of fresh fruit and vegetables, we should be able to create loose stools daily. Even those who produce a stool every day may be constipated without knowing it; if it is not easily passed and is hard and viscous then you are constipated. To correct this, simply increase your intake of dietary fibre in the form of fruit, vegetables and wholegrains. It may be advisable for those who have had constipation for some time to have enemas so that the toxic waste which has built up around the colon and bowels can be flushed out. A course of colonic irrigation with a well-qualified and experienced practitioner could also be helpful (see page 94).

OBESITY

Being severely overweight is a serious health hazard and can lead to diabetes and coronary heart disease, among other illnesses. Most people are of the opinion that obesity is caused by eating too much, but other evidence suggests that a nutritional imbalance may also be to blame. This imbalance can be caused by mixing starches and proteins or starches and fruit acids, as this reduces the absorption of nutrients.

Any attempts to lose weight quickly are dangerous and can have serious ramifications on our health. However, with food combining, the weight is lost at a steady rate. It is merely a matter of separating the 'foods that fight' and long-term weight-loss is made easy without having to count calories or deprive ourselves of food. Of course, obese people tend to eat too much anyway and we should never eat if we do not feel hungry. There is certainly a degree of truth in the saying that 'we live on a third of what we eat and the doctor lives on the other two-thirds!'

Obesity is also linked to constipation, indigestion and arthritis and the dietary advice is similar for all three – cut down drastically on refined carbohydrates such as sugar, cakes, sweets and white bread, pasta, rice, etc. and increase your intake of fruit and vegetables. Oddly enough, food combining will also help those who are underweight put on the weight that they need. This is because food combining helps the body work to its full potential so that its natural processes for maintaining body weight are working effectively. However, thin people should be warned that they too will lose weight at first.

DIABETES MELLITUS

Diabetes is a disorder of carbohydrate metabolism where sugars in the body cannot be converted into energy because the body lacks the insulin which is needed to carry out this conversion. The sugar then builds up in the bloodstream creating a state known as hyperglycaemia. If this goes untreated, then the sufferer will fall into a diabetic coma and eventually die. Diabetics do not produce enough insulin because their pancreases do not function properly so, in order to metabolise sugar, they have to inject insulin directly into the bloodstream. Conversely, hypoglycaemia comes from low blood sugar levels, and can also lead to unconsciousness. This is often caused by insulin overdose.

Those who are overweight and who repeatedly go on fad diets are prone to developing diabetes because of the strain they put on their pancreas by repeatedly starving themselves of food and then bingeing on sweet, comfort foods. There are more than 600,000 diabetics in Britain who are now officially recommended to have a diet low in fat and refined carbohydrates. The British Diabetic Association (BDA) advocates a diet which is along the same lines as food combining but with a greater emphasis on starchy foods. The BDA recommends regular meals and lots of fibre-rich foods such as fruit, vegetables and oats. The BDA also advise diabetics to cut down on fatty foods and reduce their sugar and salt intake.

ARTHRITIS

Arthritis is another incurable condition which has baffled the medical profession for years and all doctors can do is prescribe their patients anti-inflammatory drugs and painkillers. There is no single clear cause of arthritis, but there are a number of factors which are thought to lead to the development of the condition, such as injuries, abuse of the body, allergic reactions, infections, stress-exhausted adrenal glands and vitamin D deficiency. One of the causes is thought to be the accumulation of the acid end-products of digestion, so a nutritional approach to arthritis makes sense. Conventional medicine merely attempts to treat the symptoms of arthritis, ie painful, inflamed joints, but a nutritional approach tackles the cause of the condition itself. Many arthritic patients have benefited from giving up red meat, flour and sugar and adopting a diet of salads, fruit and offal, if any meat at all. Dr Hay warned that starches and sugars are the chief dietary causes of arthritis because they are usually eaten in combination with incompatible foods which interfere with their digestion. These semi-digested foods then ferment inside us, upsetting the body's chemistry and contributing to arthritis. Dr Hay advised his patients to eat acid fruits such as lemons, as they are alkaline-forming, and he also thought that celery juice was highly effective in removing years of accumulated acid deposits in the cartilage of arthritic joints. Today numerous arthritis sufferers have benefited from food combining and giving up dietary baddies such as vinegar, spices, tea, coffee and alcohol – especially sweet wines and spirits.

ALLERGY

Food combining may help to protect against allergy as it greatly improves the chemical balance of our bodies. If proteins are not digested properly they form toxic protein molecules instead of amino acids, which are their desired end-products. These toxic protein molecules contain histamine, which plays a part in many common allergies such as hay fever, asthma, migraine and eczema and is a major inflammatory agent. Dr David Munrow in his book *Man Alive, You're Half Dead!* (Bartholomew House, 1956) describes how he tested this theory on his own allergic patients. He gave them a histamine-inactivating substance (histaminase), to see how this affected their allergy after eating a mixed meal and a non-mixed meal. Dr Munrow's research revealed that his patients required more histaminase to control their symptoms when eating meals that combined carbohydrates and proteins, demonstrating that these meals produce more histamine. This is good news for the millions suffering from allergies, as eating the food-combining way may help them to control their symptoms without having to resort to antihistamine drugs, many of which cause drowsiness and most of which are expensive.

SKIN CONDITIONS

The majority of skin conditions indicate that all is not well inside the body, due to a build-up of toxins. One of the most obvious examples of this is cellulite, where toxins are stored in fatty tissues around the buttocks and thighs. Many naturopaths believe that poorly digested food ferments inside us; the body is unable to eliminate it and so stores it in fatty tissue well away from the vital organs in order to protect them. Adopting food combining will help to banish cellulite for good, as all foods will be properly digested and effectively eliminated. And the high intake of fresh fruit and vegetables will help to release the toxins which are already stored by the body, giving our insides a thorough spring-clean.

Food combining may also improve incurable conditions such as psoriasis and eczema and Dr Hay witnessed a dramatic improvement in many of his patients who suffered from these serious skin conditions. He believed that we should 'treat all skin eruptions as external evidences of internal intoxication. Set about correcting all the causes of intoxication at once, and watch the results.'

All-round Health

We have established that food combining creates an ideal chemical balance within the body and promotes better digestion, utilisation and elimination of what we put into it on a daily basis. Many ailments, such as headaches and even the common cold, have no clear cause. However, it is generally thought that a healthy body will be able to fight off a cold germ and will not be prone to developing headaches. Migraines, in particular, are interpreted by many to be a result of the body getting rid of toxins. Most migraine sufferers lose their appetite and often vomit and this is because their body is actively removing toxins. If you were to go on a detox diet, where you eat only one kind of fruit and drink only water for a few days, you would doubtless experience headaches as a result of the speedy elimination of trapped toxins.

It is certainly the case that the modern diet of processed, nutrient-deficient 'junk' food has done nothing for our general health, and the incidence of degenerative disease has never been higher. These foods do not contain the nutrients we need to maintain a healthy immune system so we can fend off illnesses, from the common cold to cancer. Diet has a major role to play in disease prevention and treatment and special research centres have been set up in the UK to monitor the effect of certain diets on fatal conditions, such as cancer. The medical profession as a whole is at last beginning to acknowledge the importance of a healthy diet and has reviewed many of the ideas that were pioneered by Dr Hay over eighty years ago.

3

Food Combining to Lose Weight

The slimming industry is huge in this country and it generates vast amounts of money. According to the Government's 1992 *Dietary and Nutritional Survey of British Adults*, 12 percent of all women and 4 percent of all men are following a rigid dieting regime at any one moment in time. That's more than seven million people! Some people are on diets of some sort throughout their entire lives and this is simply because **most diets don't work!** The plain, unpalatable truth is that short-term, fad diets simply don't lead to long-term weight-loss. The reason why these diets do not work is because they are temporary, so the results are always temporary. In fact, they are quite likely to cause more harm than good. This is because short-term dieting lasting a couple of weeks triggers the damaging 'Yo-Yo effect'. If you diet irresponsibly, the body believes it is at risk of starvation and rapidly responds by conserving energy. This leads to a lowering of our basic metabolic rate, which controls how quickly we burn our food as fuel.

The problem with lowering our metabolism is that the body adapts and learns to survive on fewer calories. Scientists have now recognised that, once the metabolism has been lowered by frugal eating, it is hard to boost it back to its previous level when the diet is stopped. During a period of intense food restriction you might only be eating around 700 calories a day, so the body becomes adept at functioning on this low calorific intake. This means that, when you return to your previous calorie intake of around 2,000 calories a day, the body stores the extra calories in the form of fat. Not only will your original weight quickly return, but you are also likely to end up feeling constantly hungry and so pile on the pounds more easily than before. This Yo-Yo rebound at the end of a period of dieting is one of the key reasons why so many diets don't work in the long term. The long-term risk factors of crash dieting followed by weight-gain may also increase the risk of heart disease and strokes.

In addition to messing up our metabolism and damaging our health, American researchers have found that being on a strict diet actually encourages fat cells to flourish! This is because, when we severely restrict our eating, the body protects itself against possible famine by actually storing more fat. Very low-calorie diets simply increase the efficiency of fat storage, so extreme restriction of eating boosts unwanted fat cells! While this does not mean that we can lose weight by living on cream cakes and chips, it does show that long-term successful slimming requires a change in tactics from conventional calorie counting.

One of the reasons why food combining helps us to lose weight and keep it off *permanently* is because it is a long-term eating plan. The philosophy of food combining is also very different from that of diets that encourage us continuously to deprive ourselves of food. Food deprivation tends to create the wrong mentality, where we think of food as our enemy instead of the essential source of energy and vitality that it is. Food combining allows us to eat as much food as we like as long as it is the right kind of food, and this will help us to lose weight forever! Of course, if you take up food combining temporarily, then your weight-loss will only be temporary, but if you adopt it as a permanent eating plan, then the results will be permanent. Do not expect to lose weight suddenly with food combining; food combining helps us to lose weight steadily and this is a healthier way to shed excess weight.

Many of the so-called 'fad diets' are also too regimented (or too ridiculous) to be adopted in the long term. One may recommend that we eat nothing but banana milkshakes, another will recommend lots of steaks and red wine and yet another will favour carbohydrates and nothing else. Many of these fad diets not only upset our digestive system and metabolism, but are also unhealthy and deprive our bodies of vital nutrients.

The good thing about food combining is that there is no tiresome calorie counting. A healthy adult needs a daily supply of around 1,800–2,500 kilocalories, so those who are on strict diets of only 700–800 kilocalories a day are depriving themselves of the nutrients and energy that they need, as well as slowing down their metabolism. With food combining you can eat tasty, sustaining meals that give your body all the nutrients it needs. It is important to bear in mind that your natural body weight will not necessarily be that of an excessively slim super model! Many of these girls survive on a steady diet of cigarettes and champagne and little else. There is no doubt that if you strive to acquire the anorexic look, you will be depriving your body of vital nutrients and damaging your health.

Hypoglycaemia

Dieting can be bad for your health and it is not uncommon for dieters to experience headaches, dizziness, palpitations, anxiety, poor coordination, energy loss, extreme coldness, excessive perspiration, drowsiness and other unpleasant symptoms. This is often caused by a condition known as hypoglycaemia, where the levels of glucose in the blood fluctuate dramatically and fall way below normal levels. When this happens, dieters feel the sudden urge to eat something immediately, usually sweet, and this is why many dieters follow the constant pattern of food deprivation followed by bingeing on sweet snacks.

Hypoglycaemic cravings should not be ignored! They exist because the body knows that very low blood glucose is dangerous and can lead to diabetes, coma and even death. All diabetics can experience hypoglycaemic attacks and they learn how to deal with them effectively. In emergency situations, where there is no other food around, something sweet should be eaten, although this solution is not advised for all attacks, and certainly not if insulin deprivation is suspected. However, many dieters resort to this remedy continuously, unaware of the fact that they are becoming dependent upon a dangerously addictive drug. Sweet food increases the blood glucose level to such an extent that insulin is produced by the pancreas to bring the blood glucose level back under control. However, in dieters who often deal with their hypoglycaemia by eating sweet foods, the pancreas can become 'trigger happy' and send too much of the hormone into the blood. This causes the glucose level to fall dramatically and so a vicious circle is formed. If this happens too often, pancreatic insulin production may break down altogether, causing diabetes.

Food combining wipes out this problem because it encourages us to eat substantial meals which will keep our blood glucose levels normal for hours. Hunger pangs between meals should vanish but, if you do feel hungry, then you should not deprive yourself of food. Some feel the need to eat little and often and it is fine to snack on neutral foods (see the table in Chapter 5). Here are some tips to keep mood swings and other symptoms of hypoglycaemia at bay:

* Always eat something for breakfast. It is best to have only raw fresh fruit on its own or mixed with some live yoghurt, but if you feel that this is not enough to keep you going, you can have a more substantial breakfast of porridge and a banana.

* If you are hungry between meals, snack on fresh fruit, raisins, dried apricots, or seeds. All of these can be bought from health-food shops and good supermarkets.

* You may find that you need to eat little and often to conserve your energy levels, and there is nothing wrong with this as long as you do not mix starches and proteins in the space of three or four hours.

* Try to make lunch your biggest meal as the energy from the food will keep you going through the remainder of the day.

* If you are hungry at bedtime, have a few rye biscuits (starch) or some natural yoghurt (protein). If you wake up with night sweats, it could be because your blood glucose levels are too low.

* Avoid eating 'quick release' sugars such as chocolates, cakes and sweets, and strong chemicals like caffeine and alcohol.

* Stress affects the body in many ways – it can contribute to hypoglycaemic attacks. Try to relax and make sure that you are getting enough sleep.

* If you find it impossible to resist the urge to eat something sweet, then you can eat honey, real maple syrup, blackstrap molasses or real sugar, but do not eat food containing ordinary white or brown sugar. All sweetenings are acid forming, with the exception of blackstrap molasses, which is seen as neutral. As an alternative to chocolate try carob, a tasty vegetable substitute which is available in a powder and in bar form. It is an excellent alternative to chocolate and contains no caffeine. Carob should be listed under carbohydrates.

Eating to Lose Weight

Storing toxins internally can also be responsible for weight-gain. All our cells are continually renewed and this means that old discarded cells will eventually ferment and turn toxic if the body is unable to eliminate them. As we have seen, poorly digested food also turns toxic in the body and, if these two types of waste are not effectively eliminated every day, then a build-up occurs and this is usually stored in our fat cells well away from the vital organs. In addition, these toxins are acidic, so our bodies retain water to neutralise the acid, giving us a bloated appearance. This build-up of trapped toxins can grow every day and will have a cumulative effect on our body until it can eliminate the food effectively. However, if we continue to hamper our digestive processes by eating processed food and protein and carbohydrates together at meals, this store of toxic waste will grow and our weight will continue to soar, or at least we will find it very difficult to lose weight.

The food-combining meal planner outlined in Chapter 5 lists mainly fruit and vegetables which have a very high water content. This means that we can eat as much as we like of these foods without putting on any weight. Humans comprise a staggering 70 percent water and so, to maintain a healthy body, we need to continuously replenish our supplies of water. It makes sense, therefore, to eat foods which are high in water. Drinking gallons of pure water every day will not have the same effect, although it will help to flush out toxins from the body. Other foods are concentrated, meaning that the water content has been removed, either through processing or through cooking. The most healthy and effective way of losing weight is by adopting a diet that is 70 percent fruit and vegetables and only 30 percent concentrated foods such as grains, meat, fish and legumes (pulses).

The reason why the water present in fruit and vegetables is so beneficial is because it transports the nutrients in the fruit to the body cells that need them, as well as helping to flush away the toxins and waste inside us. Nearly all our nutritional requirements are met by eating fruit and vegetables which are rich in vitamins, minerals, amino acids (proteins), fibre, enzymes, carbohydrates and fatty acids. If you do not eat enough of these vital foods, you are not feeding your body the essential nutrients that it needs to carry out all its processes effectively. Even if you are taking a daily vitamin supplement, there is no guarantee that your body is able to make use of these nutrients as effectively as it does with the nutrients that are naturally present in food. In order to feel alive and healthy, it is important to eat foods that are also alive and healthy and eating fresh fruit and vegetables is the answer.

In the wild, animals do not suffer from the same degenerative illnesses or obesity that many humans fall victim to. This is partly because they do not have a diet of highly processed, refined foods, but live off uncooked food with a high water content. Other mammals eat to live, whereas we humans are more interested in satisfying our taste buds than making sure that we eat the right foods.

We need to adopt the diet of our forebears if we are to attain good health and slim figures. Making high water-content foods 70 percent of our daily diet is not as difficult and restricting as it may seem. A breakfast of fruit salad will take you halfway there. Then, making sure that you have sufficient vegetables with your lunch and dinner will provide the required amount. However, it may be slightly more difficult to maintain this balance of food every day, especially if you are out and about and are unable to make your own meals. If so, then do not feel guilty about it! Simply make up for all the concentrated foods that you have eaten on a bad day by eating predominantly raw fruit and vegetables the following day. Soon you will see your excess weight disappear and you won't have to deprive yourself of food in the process.

Food Combining to Gain Weight?

Strange as it may seem, food combining can also help those who are very thin to put on weight. Some people eat vast amounts of food but find it impossible to reach an ideal weight. This may be due to a number of factors such as recent illness, consumption of energy and metabolic rate. For these people, the desire to put on weight is just as strong as the desire in others to lose it. Those who need to put on weight often adopt an unhealthy, high-fat diet of sweets, biscuits and cakes to pile on the pounds while cutting down on all the good food such as fruit and vegetables, but this does not help them in their quest, whereas food combining can. The body cannot make use of these processed foods, but with food combining each meal is more effectively digested and assimilated and so the body is better nourished. Only when the body is properly nourished can it reach its healthy weight.

—— 4 ——

The Food Groups Explained

In order to combine the right foods successfully, we need to take a closer look at the different food groups: protein, carbohydrate, neutral foods, fruit and herbs and spices.

Protein

Many of us worry about whether we are getting enough protein in our diet, but few think to question whether we are eating too much protein or stop to wonder which sources of protein are best. Expert views on this particular food group vary dramatically; some say that our diet should consist mostly of protein, while others insist that it should be kept to a minimum. Protein is perhaps the most complicated of all nutrients and its assimilation and utilisation by the body is an equally complicated procedure. We do not simply produce protein when we eat protein-rich foods. Protein is built from the amino acids in food and all the different sources of protein contain these amino acid building-blocks. For example, animal protein is different from human protein and, when we eat meat, the protein must first be split into its component amino acids before we can create the protein that we need from it. Therefore, the value of protein-rich food lies in its amino acids.

There are twenty-three different amino acids and fifteen of these can be produced by the body. The body must obtain the other eight from another source and so these are termed 'essential'. Believe it or not, all these essential amino acids can be obtained from eating vegetables, nuts, wholegrains, seeds or sprouts regularly and we do not have to eat meat or animal products at all. Very few people suffer from protein deficiency and, contrary to widespread opinion, we do not need to eat a great deal of protein in order to survive. What is more, our bodies recycle 70 percent of the waste from protein and keep stores of all the various amino acids. This constant supply of amino acids is known as the amino acid pool. When the body needs protein, it simply takes the amino acids from the lymph and blood and builds the protein it needs. When the amino acid pool contains plenty of amino acids, the liver absorbs and stores them until the body requires them.

WHICH PROTEIN SOURCE IS BEST?

It has been impressed on most of us that meat is a vital source of protein and, without it, our bodies would be seriously lacking, but this simply is not true. In fact, we generally eat far more protein than our bodies need and we can easily obtain sufficient protein from a good mix of cereals and vegetables. Whether we eat protein in the form of meat, cereals or vegetables, it has to be broken down into the various amino acids, which are then reassembled to form human protein.

Although some health writers and advocates of the Hay system suggest that vegetables are a better source of protein than meat, this is not the view prevailing among qualified nutritionists who maintain that protein from animal sources is closest to human protein. Egg and milk protein are thought to be closest to human requirements. Again, some health writers assert that protein is destroyed by various cooking processes, in which case meat protein would be ruined. However, Dr Anne Walker asserts that 'the majority of amino acids are fairly robust and cooking meat does not destroy the amino acids present, although there may be some alteration around the edge of food which has been subjected to extreme heat, as in an oven.' In fact, cooking can sometimes make the amino acids more accessible to the body. Dr Walker explains, 'In the case of seeds, the protein present is locked in globules which are inaccessible to our enzymes. However, cooking the seeds opens up the protein which can then be utilised by the body.

Although meat is a valuable source of protein, there is no doubt that we can live without it and obtain the protein we need from cereal and vegetable sources. These foods are also healthier and more nutritious than meat which contains saturated fat, a substance of little nutritional value that is thought to contribute to the development of heart disease. All in all, vegetables and wholegrains are a far healthier source of protein and you will be getting plenty when food combining.

EAT LESS PROTEIN TO LOSE WEIGHT

Our bodies lose only 23g of protein a day through faeces, urine, hair, dead skin and perspiration. To replace this you would only need to eat a pound and a half of protein a month. The majority of us eat far more protein than we actually need and this puts a heavy burden on the system. We use considerable energy in trying to eliminate this excess of protein, energy which could be better used by the body. The excess protein not only consumes our energy supplies, it also gets stored in the body as toxic waste which can cause us to put on weight and may lead to the development of cellulite!

Protein digestion itself is very complicated and our bodies use a great deal of energy in the process. This means that, when protein digestion is disrupted by eating carbohydrates at the same meal, the level of waste from protein is higher. It can take as long as twenty-five hours, sometimes even days, for meat to pass through our long and twisted digestive system. During this time, the meat putrefies and emits toxins. This often results in bad breath, body odour, excessive sweating and foul-smelling stools which are all signs that the body is doing its best to eliminate the toxic waste from meat. At the other end of the scale is fruit, which is digested very quickly and, if you switch to a diet of only raw fruit and vegetables, you should experience none of these unpleasant symptoms.

PROTEIN FOODS
Meat (acid-forming)
Whether you are food combining to lose weight or to boost your health, factory-farmed beef or pork and battery-raised poultry are best avoided. In these conditions, the animals are fed growth hormones, antibiotics and other chemicals that only add to the burden of toxic waste inside us instead of helping to reduce it. If you are a real meat fan, then the best meats to eat are lamb, as they are usually allowed to roam free, and free-range poultry. Organically reared beef and pork is also not as hard to find as it used to be, so ask your local butcher if they have any genuinely organic meat.

Fish (acid-forming)
Fish is a healthier source of protein than meat. It contains less fat and the fat it does contain is of the beneficial, polyunsaturated kind. In fact, fish oil is extremely good for us and is an excellent source of vitamins A and D and essential fatty acids. Buy fresh fish and cook it within twenty-four hours. Some frozen fish is sprayed with chemical preservatives and the packaging does not indicate this. Processed fish, ie salted and smoked, should also be avoided as processing destroys much of the nutrients that are present in the fish in its natural state and the processes themselves involve chemical treatments.

Eggs (acid-forming)
Eggs are a rich source of protein but, like all animal products,

they are also high in saturated fat. Always use free-range eggs as those from battery-reared hens will probably contain artificial colours and additives and, apart from anything else, free-range eggs taste better and involve less cruelty to the hens.

Cheese (acid-forming)

All cheeses, no matter what animal they come from, are protein foods, although some cream cheeses contain a very low amount of protein, and are compatible with carbohydrates. If you wish to lose weight, you should try to give up cheese, except for very low-fat varieties such as cottage cheese. All processed cheeses should also be avoided as they tend to contain artificial preservatives such as nitrates (read the labels before you buy).

Milk (acid- and alkali-forming)

This complete protein is both acid-forming and alkaline-forming, depending upon the form in which the milk is consumed. In its raw, unpasteurised state it is alkaline-forming, but it becomes more acid-forming the more it is heat treated. This means that most of the milk we buy in cartons and bottles is acid-forming. In general, milk does not combine well with other foods and it is very mucus forming, which can cause trouble with our sinuses. The milk produced by each species of animal is designed to feed that particular species alone. This helps to explain why infants fed on breast milk tend not to suffer from the symptoms of intolerance that some babies fed on cow's milk experience. Many people are intolerant to cow's milk and suffer from constant sinus problems as a result, because their bodies lack the enzymes to digest it. When cow's milk is mixed with other foods it is even more difficult to digest as it interferes with the digestion of both proteins and carbohydrates. Those who do have an intolerance to cow's milk may find that they can cope better with goat's or sheep's milk, but these should not be mixed with other foods either.

Soya milk really is not milk at all, but a white liquid made from soya beans. It does not taste like cow's milk but some do use it as a substitute. However, it is a processed product and the protein molecules in soya milk are very large, bigger than in cow's milk, and so put extra strain on our overworked digestive systems.

Yoghurt (alkaline-forming)
Surprisingly, yoghurt is alkaline-forming and it is a great source of protein. Standard yoghurt is made with pasteurised, full-fat milk; low-fat yoghurts are made with skimmed milk; and 'bio' or 'live' yoghurt contain live cultures of the friendly bacteria *Streptococcus lactus* and *Streptococcus thermophilus*. Yoghurt is easier to digest than milk, as the milk sugar lactose is broken down into lactic acid by the yoghurt culture. However, not all yoghurts are healthy – many are heat treated in sterilisation processes and their natural culture is destroyed. These yoghurts are believed to be acid-forming and are best avoided. Although yoghurt is a protein, it can be mixed occasionally with oats to make muesli (see Chapter 6).

Carbohydrates

Carbohydrates, or starches, provide the energy we need to carry out all our bodily processes. Starch foods include wheat and grains such as bread, pasta and rice and also some fruit and vegetables, such as potatoes and bananas. We need to eat these foods in order to get the energy we need, and some of us will need more than others. For example, athletes need to eat a copious amount of carbohydrate to replenish the energy they burn off in exercise. Those who are not so active do not need to eat as much carbohydrate, and remember – excess carbohydrate is stored by the body as **fat!**

When asked to name a carbohydrate, bread would probably be the first food to come to mind, as we seem to eat more bread, and wheat products in general, than anything else. Good quality bread is a valuable source of fibre, but much of the bread available in our supermarkets is made by an industrial method involving double the amount of yeast (a common cause of food intolerance) for rapid fermentation. Many of these loaves also contain 'improvers' and other additives, such as monoacetyltartaric acid and chlorine dioxide. The manufacturers attempt to baffle us further by labelling some breads as 'brown' when, in fact, these have just been disguised with an artificial colouring. Bread and other wheat products can also aggravate mucus production, as can milk and dairy products. Processed varieties of bread are severely mucus-forming and should be avoided by anyone who suffers from sinus problems, catarrh and digestive or bowel disorders. For more information on food intolerance and food allergies, read my *Quick Guide to Food Allergies* (Boxtree, 1995, £3.99).

However, if you are intolerant to wheat and its derivatives, there are numerous other sources of carbohydrate, and some of them are easier for our bodies to digest than wheat. These include oats, rye, buckwheat, millet, potatoes, rice and many more grains. It is better for us to eat wholegrains as these are easier for the body to digest. This means eating wholemeal bread, brown rice and wholemeal pasta. With the exception of millet, all grains are acid-forming.

WHEAT AND OTHER GRAINS

Wheat is Britain's most important crop and, not surprisingly, our diet is dominated by it. All wheat products, such as bread and pasta, have a high gluten content and large numbers of us are mildly intolerant to gluten with symptoms such as diarrhoea, anaemia due to poor iron absorption, tiredness, skin rashes and recurrent mouth ulcers. However, it is possible to find wheat products which do not have such a high gluten content, like rye bread.

Wheat bran

Wheat bran is *not* the best fibre provider, although many food manufacturers spend a great deal of airtime trying to convince us that it is. Wheat bran certainly deserves the title 'roughage' as that is exactly what it is: harsh, rough and difficult to digest. In fact, wheat bran irritates the sensitive colon wall and often causes food intolerance and bowel disorders. This can result in poor elimination of waste – contrary to what most of us are led to believe.

Cracked wheat, or bulgar

This is a processed wheat product made from broken grains. The most nutritious way to eat cracked wheat is presoaked and it can be used to make a delicious salad dish called Tabbouleh (see Chapter 6).

Semolina

This is the grittiest part of durum wheat, sifted out and made into hardened pasta products.

Wholewheat

This is made from the wholewheat kernel and it is the best way to enjoy wheat.

Barley

This is one of the key ingredients in bread baking today. Unrefined barley (pot barley) has high levels of iron, calcium, potassium and B vitamins (notably folic acid) and it can help to soothe the stomach, digestive and urinary tracts. Pot barley should be soaked overnight before using, but keep the soaking water for cooking as it will contain important vitamins. It takes about an hour to cook pot barley and it is a delicious addition to rice dishes.

Buckwheat
Despite its name, buckwheat is totally gluten-free and nothing like our common wheat. It actually comes from a small plant related to rhubarb. Buckwheat contains B vitamins, potassium, magnesium and iron as well as the eight essential amino acids. Buckwheat grouts can be washed and cooked in the same way as rice, and buckwheat flour can be used in baking recipes and to thicken sauces and soups.

Basmati rice
This comes from the foothills of the Himalayas and is a fine, long-grain rice. It has a lovely aromatic flavour but is not as healthy as brown rice.

Brown rice
This is the entire rice pellet, including its protective bran coating, and is an excellent source of fibre. Brown rice also contains iron, calcium, B vitamins and many essential amino acids.

Maize
This is a versatile, gluten-free grain and can be eaten whole in the form of corn-on-the-cob, served as sweet corn, or ground into cornflour.

Millet
One of the great benefits of millet is that it has the same high protein content as wheat but without the sticky gluten that goes with it. It also contains more iron than other cereals and is a useful source of calcium. Millet can be used as an alternative to rice but 'crack' the tiny seeds first by frying them in a little olive

oil, as this helps them to absorb enough cooking water to become soft.

Oats

Oats are an important staple food and contain protein, B vitamins and even the healthy polyunsaturated fats. Porridge is an excellent energy-giving breakfast and oats are also a good base for healthy snacks such as flapjacks. Oatbran has also been shown to regulate blood sugar levels and may even help diabetics as it encourages insulin stability.

Rye

Rye has a similar composition to wheat but has a low gluten content. Many who find themselves allergic to wheat and its products, such as bread, can eat rye bread as an alternative.

Sago

Sago comes in dry granules obtained from the sago palm. It is very easily digested, has no allergy-associated problems and is traditionally used for making milk puddings for invalids. Although bland and lacking in fibre, sago is useful for those on a restricted or gluten-free diet.

AN EXCEPTION TO THE RULE

Both bananas and potatoes in their skins are alkaline-forming, but they are classed as carbohydrates because they are at least 20 percent starch. This means that you should not mix them with protein foods – so no more meat and potatoes! The best way to reap the benefits of potatoes, such as their high vitamin C content, is to eat them baked with the skins on. Due to the anti-sprouting chemicals that are sprayed onto potatoes, it is best to buy organically grown varieties. Baked potatoes are very low in calories and make a tasty and substantial meal with some butter and salad.

PULSES – A FOOD COMBINING CONUNDRUM

Pulses or legumes include beans, lentils, peas, chick peas and peanuts. They do not easily slot into the food-combining jigsaw as they have high concentrations of both starch and protein. Dr Hay classified them as starch and thought that they were best avoided, but many beans are a rich source of protein. Pulses are acid-forming and they are generally believed to be responsible for wreaking havoc on our digestive systems. They do not combine well with either proteins or carbohydrates and are renowned for causing flatulence, hence the jokes about baked beans. Soya beans and soya products such as tofu, tempeh, miso, soya flour and soya milk are all concentrated proteins. They cause digestive problems in some of us and are best avoided.

However, many pulses are a valuable source of protein for vegetarians as well as being rich in iron, calcium, zinc, magnesium and B vitamins. If they are properly prepared and not combined with proteins or starches then they are far less likely to cause digestive upsets. It has also been discovered that the fibre present in pulses can help to control the level of blood glucose and is recommended for diabetics and hypoglycaemics. What is more, according to nutritionist Kathryn Marsden, pulses can help to create butyric acid which is formed during the breakdown of dietary fibre.

Sprouted pulses

By far the best way to eat pulses is when they are sprouted. This can easily be done at home, by soaking and then leaving the beans on a damp tea cloth on the window sill or in an airing cupboard. Most grains, beans and seeds can be sprouted this way and this increases their vitamin, mineral and enzyme levels dramatically, as well as converting the starch into natural sugars. The most successful varieties of pulses for sprouting are alfalfa, lentils and mung beans. They are delicious eaten raw in salads or simply sprinkled with a little freshly squeezed lemon juice.

SUGAR

Refined sugar is one of the biggest dietary baddies, particularly refined white sugar. It does us absolutely no good whatsoever and is, in fact, linked to obesity and diabetes as well as mental disturbances such as hyperactivity and even violent behaviour. Our consumption of refined sugar has increased dramatically since the 1960s with the huge variety of sweets, cakes and biscuits which are now available. Sugar is also added to most processed foods from baked beans to chicken curry, so look carefully on packaging to check for this. The only sugar we need is the natural sugar present in fruit, and refined sugar and all other refined carbohydrates should be avoided.

Neutral Foods

The title 'neutral' does not mean that the foods in this list have a neutral pH balance; they may be either acid- or alkaline-forming. It simply means that these foods mix well with both carbohydrates and proteins and also combine well with each other.

VEGETABLES

Vegetables and salads are alkaline-forming and you can have them in abundance with both protein and carbohydrate meals. Due to modern farming methods, it is best to use organically grown vegetables which have not been sprayed with toxic pesticides, herbicides and fungicides. Much of the fruit and vegetables we get in the UK are imported and we have no idea of what chemicals are used in their cultivation. If you cannot get hold of organically grown fruit and vegetables, then make sure you either remove the skins or scrub them thoroughly with soapy water. A startling amount of dirt, bacteria and chemical residues can be removed by thorough cleaning.

Nuts

Most nuts are acid-forming except for almonds and Brazils. Nuts are a highly concentrated food and should only be eaten in small amounts with starch and protein meals. Nuts are best combined with salads and there are a couple of tasty nut salad recipes in Chapter 6. If you are trying to lose weight, then you may wish to avoid nuts altogether as they are a rich source of polyunsaturated oils which are very good for us healthwise, but are high in calories. Many dieters make the mistake of trying to cut fat completely from their diet, but we do need a certain amount of fat to produce healthy cells. Always eat nuts slowly so that they can be broken up in the mouth where the process of digestion begins. Avoid processed nuts, ie salted or dry roasted varieties.

Seeds

Seeds are alkaline-forming and are rich in vitamins, minerals and essential fatty acids. However, seeds turn rancid if they are not properly stored. They are best kept in an airtight container in the refrigerator. In general, seeds are easy to digest and are great to snack on.

Fats and oils

Fats and oils are neutral, so they can be used in both protein and carbohydrate meals. We all need fats in our diet, but it is important to distinguish between the different types of fat. The body needs essential fatty acids to carry out many of its processes and these are found in polyunsaturated oils (from vegetables, nuts, seeds and fish) such as olive oil and cod liver oil. Some of these oils are better for cooking purposes than others, as heat degrades some oils. When oil is heated above 100°C (212°F) it not only wipes out important nutrients, but also generates free radicals into the bargain. These destructive molecular fragments have been implicated in all kinds of health scares, from heart disease to cancer and premature ageing. Nature has cleverly equipped oils with vitamin E. This is an antioxidant which protects oil against rancidity and neutralises free radicals. Unfortunately, vitamin E is also destroyed by heat. However, some oils are more stable than others during cooking – olive oil is best. This nutritious oil is monounsaturated, the healthiest type, and it also makes delicious salad dressings.

BUTTER OR MARGARINE?

There is so much confusion and controversy surrounding what we should be spreading on our bread that it is well worth taking a quick look at the issues involved. Butter is relatively high in saturated fat but is still a natural product, whereas margarines and low-fat spreads are highly processed products made with complicated chemical wizardry. Although low-fat margarines contain healthy polyunsaturates and are low in saturates, the oil has been through a process known as hydrogenation and this changes the structure of the oil, making it behave in the body as if it were a saturated fat. Many nutritionists are now of the opinion that the hydrogenation process is hazardous to our health as it creates trans-fats. These may, in the long term, contribute to coronary heart disease.

For these reasons, this *Quick Guide* recommends the use of olive oil and butter in cooking and spreading. However, all fats are very high in calories and should be kept to a minimum if you are trying to lose weight, although they should not be avoided entirely. Another consideration is that, when large amounts of fat are mixed with protein, digestion of the protein is hindered. If you would rather use a healthy, low-fat alternative to butter, then try unhydrogenated spreads, found in health-food stores.

Again, it should be stressed that you must *not* exclude fat completely from your diet as you will also be cutting out the important essential fatty acids. One of the most important essential fatty acids is linoleic acid which comes from polyun-saturated vegetable oils. Essential fatty acids form part of every cell in the body and they are needed for a wide range of processes. Signs of fat deficiency are arthritis, nervous disorders and skin problems.

CREAM
Single, whipping, double and even clotted cream are allowed with any foods! So if you want a sweet treat, why not have some banana and fresh cream? However, if you want to lose weight, bear in mind that cream is very high in calories and fat, so is best avoided.

HERBS AND SPICES
There are thousands of aromatic herbs and spices, such as basil, oregano, coriander and mint, which add a great deal of flavour to our cooking. Herbs and spices are neutral and can be eaten in abundance with all foods, which is just as well considering how bland our meals would be without them. Herbs, when fresh, are packed with nutrients and have been used for centuries in cooking and beauty therapies and in the treatment of numerous ailments.

Fruits and Fruit Juices

Fresh fruit and their juices are alkali-forming and they are the easiest foods for our body to digest, assimilate and eliminate. In fact, an apple takes only about fifteen minutes to pass through the stomach, whereas a heavy protein meal will take at least five hours. Fruit is a great fibre provider and it contains a wealth of vitamins and minerals. It is also 70 percent water and very low in calories and so is ideal for flushing out the internal system and aiding weight-loss. With food combining, we should eat one totally alkaline meal a day and breakfast is often the best time for this. A fresh fruit salad is the best way to start the day. Up until midday our bodies are still in their elimination mode and eating fruit will boost these processes. Fruit is also rich in enzymes, which assist in their digestion. Some fruit, such as apples, also contain a substance called pectin which aids the removal of toxins.

However, it is not so good for us to eat fruit as a dessert. Fruit is designed to go straight through our digestive system and so it is best eaten on an empty stomach. It is then easily digested without using up any energy that may be needed to eliminate toxins and break down fat. If you eat an apple after a protein meal, the fruit will either speed up the passage of protein, which is then made to leave the stomach before it is properly digested, or the protein will cause the fruit to stay too long in the stomach so that it starts to ferment. Neither event is desirable as both poorly digested protein and rotten fruit just add to our store of toxins and can cause indigestion pains.

ACID FRUITS

Contrary to what this suggests, acid fruits are not acid-forming at all. Under this heading come grapefruit, oranges, lemons, blackberries, etc. These fruits do, indeed, have an acid taste, but this should not be confused with their end-product, which is alkaline. The acids in these fruits actually leave the body about an hour after they have been eaten, primarily through the four main organs of elimination: the lungs, skin, urinary tract and bowels. Lemon, which most people think of as particularly acidic, is actually very good for detoxing our insides. A slice of lemon in hot water is a good drink to have first thing in the morning and late at night to help stimulate our processes of elimination. Acid fruits should not be mixed with starches at the same meal.

STEWED FRUIT

Dr Hay believed that stewed fruits are 'dead fruits' and for optimum health we should be eating as much 'live' food as possible. Heat changes the chemical status of fruit, making it more acidic and destroying many of its important vitamins and enzymes. Prunes and rhubarb are not allowed in this food-combining diet as they contain oxalic acid, which is hard to digest and binds with minerals so that they cannot be utilised by the body.

DRIED FRUIT

Dried fruits are also alkaline-forming and they mix well with each other, but should not be mixed with protein or starch. Most dried fruit is sprayed with glazing agents and sulphur dioxide preservatives and these are best avoided – so check on the packaging. You can buy additive-free dried fruit from health food stores. Raisins and dried apricots are great to snack on and they help to stimulate bowel movements.

Study the table on the following page to see at a glance the foods that are alkaline-forming and those that are acid-forming (remember a balanced diet should consist of 25 percent acid-forming and 75 percent alkali-forming food):

Acid-forming food	Alkali-forming food
barley	almonds
beans	brazil nuts
bread	chestnuts
breakfast cereals	fruits
buckwheat	hazelnuts
cashew nuts	millet
cheese	pine kernels
chick peas	vegetables
eggs	
fish	
flour	
game	
meat	
oats	
peanuts	
peas (dried)	
pecan nuts	
poultry	
rice	
sugar	
walnuts	
wheat and wheat products	

5

Successful Food Combining

One of the best things about food combining is that the emphasis is on fresh foods, so many of the meal suggestions and recipes require very little cooking with no compromise on taste. The meals are quick to make, flexible and interchangeable and are perfect for those who lead busy lives or for those who simply do not want to spend too much time in the kitchen. As soon as you get to know the different food groups, you will be able to combine the right foods without a second's thought. Until then, study the table below to discover at a glance which foods are protein, carbohydrate or neutral. The foods in the left column must *not* be mixed with the foods in the right column. The neutral foods in the central column can be mixed with the foods in the left and right columns:

Protein	Neutral	Carbohydrate
cheese	butter	biscuits
eggs	cream	bread
fish	herbs	cakes
meat	oils	crackers
milk	nuts	sweet fruits *
poultry	salads	honey
shellfish	seeds	maple syrup
soya beans	spreads	millet
soya products	vegetables except	maize (corn)
yoghurt	potatoes, sweet	oats

Protein	Neutral	Carbohydrate
	potatoes	pasta
		pastry
		potatoes
		rice
		sugar
		sweet potatoes
		sweets

* *such as custard apples, dates, figs, extra-sweet grapes, papaya and pears (if very sweet and ripe).*

Your Shopping List

It is a good idea to make sure that your cupboards and fridge are full of the fresh ingredients you need to make food combining easy. Apart from bounteous amounts of fresh fruit and vegetables, there are other foods which are the basis for tasty, healthy meals:

* brown rice
* extra virgin olive oil – the healthiest oil there is!
* free-range eggs
* dried fruit – raisins, sultanas and dried figs (these are all great for snacking on and for making fruit compote)
* garlic and other herbs (preferably fresh), such as basil, bay leaves, coriander, fennel, oregano, parsley, peppermint, rosemary, tarragon and thyme
* black pepper and sea salt for seasoning
* oatbran, oatmeal or oatgerm
* nuts – Brazils, almonds, pecans, pinenuts and walnuts
* seeds – pumpkin seeds, sunflower seeds and linseeds
* soy or tamari sauce
* wholewheat bread

* wholegrain crackers
* wholewheat pasta
* cracked wheat
* millet
* pot barley
* free-range poultry
* fresh fish
* wholegrain mustard
* alternatives to ordinary granulated sugar: blackstrap molasses, organic unblended honey, natural maple syrup, fructose (fruit sugar – useful for baking and is twice as sweet as ordinary sugar and so half the amount is needed).

It is important to read all food labelling carefully to see what chemicals have been added, and choose organically grown food wherever possible and free-range chicken and eggs.

Our Aim

Remember that every day we should aim to have:

* one wholly alkaline meal
* one protein meal
* one carbohydrate meal.

To achieve this aim, it is easier to have the alkaline meal in the morning, when our stomachs do not demand much. Then at lunch-time we can either have a protein or starch meal and in the evening we can have whichever food group was avoided at lunch. These basic rules of food combining are easy to remember and soon you will know exactly what to eat and at what time. However, you must not punish yourself and, if you start the day with all good intentions by having a fresh fruit breakfast, but feel ravenously hungry at 11am, do not deprive yourself of food. If you are hungry, have some fruit or nuts (see the section on snacks on pages 68–9). Similarly, if, for whatever reason, you eat mainly concentrated foods on one day, then simply make up for this by eating mainly fresh fruit and vegetables the following day. Here are some basic tips for successful food combining:

* Never mix concentrated proteins and carbohydrates
* Try to eat only one type of protein at each protein meal and only one type of starch at each carbohydrate meal
* Neutral foods can be mixed with both carbohydrates and proteins
* Use refined or cold-pressed vegetable oils such as sunflower, corn, olive, soya or wheatgerm, which are all high in polyunsaturates. Fry vegetables only very lightly in hot olive oil to preserve their goodness
* Use butter instead of margarine, but use it in moderation if you are trying to lose weight
* Always look for fresh, quality food when shopping, preferably organic, as this will contain less chemical pesticides and hormones than produce which is farmed using modern methods
* Try to have more vegetables with each meal and cut down on concentrated starch and protein. For example, if you are having lamb chops and courgettes as a meal, limit yourself to one lamb chop, but go mad on the courgettes in butter and garlic
* Avoid all refined and processed foods
* Try to fill up on your main meals so that you can leave a gap of four hours until you next eat something
* Cut down on the amount of salt you use in your cooking, and use only sea salt

* Cut down on the amount of sugar you eat, and if you need something sweet use blackstrap molasses, honey, real maple syrup or crystallised ginger
* Instead of frying meat, poultry or fish, cook them gently in a covered pan in their own juices, grill them or roast them in the oven.

Low-energy Foods

One of the aims of food combining is to cut out *low-energy* foods because they are not life-giving foods. Here, 'energy' does not refer to calories but to nutritional value and, in fact, low-energy foods tend to be high in calories but can actually sap our energy because the body finds them difficult to digest and metabolise. Low-energy foods are:

* artificial sweeteners
* artificial colours, flavours and preservatives
* white and brown sugar
* sweets and chocolate
* coffee, tea, cocoa, cola, hot chocolate
* alcohol
* pasteurised orange juice
* most polyunsaturated spreads
* processed 'low-fat' foods
* tap water
* cow's milk and soya milk
* pizzas, pastries, pies and refined pasta
* salt
* salty snacks such as salted peanuts
* beef, pork and related products
* battery-raised poultry and their eggs
* processed, smoked and coloured cheeses

* burned food
* deep-fried foods
* white flour and bread.

Foods to Avoid

Here is a more detailed list of the nutrient-deficient foods that we should avoid on the food-combining diet:

All refined carbohydrates. This means sugar in all forms, except blackstrap molasses, real maple syrup, honey, crystallised ginger or fructose. Also avoid carbonated soft drinks, flavoured squashes and all bottled fruit drinks, as these are high in sugar. White flour and white-flour products should also be avoided, including white bread, white polished rice and other refined grains such as sago and tapioca. Cakes, biscuits, pastries and puddings made from white flour should be cut out of your diet. Many good-quality bakers and supermarkets sell cakes made with wholemeal flour, but it is best to make your own so you can ensure that all the ingredients are as wholesome as possible.

Desserts, puddings and sugary foods are usually made from starch and protein; a mixture of flour, eggs and milk as well as lots of unhealthy sugar. They should therefore be avoided, but the odd treat is not going to harm you and you can always make up for this later by eating more fresh fruit and vegetables.

Most processed foods and ready-made meals should be avoided because of all the colourings, flavourings, preservatives and stabilisers that these foods contain to give them flavour and a long shelf-life. All synthetic additives have to undergo rigorous testing, but the long-term effects of consuming high levels of these additives is as yet unknown. In the short term, some food additives are thought to cause hyperactivity in children, particularly food dyes. My daughter's behaviour goes rapidly downhill after just one Smartie! There are many different groups of additives: flavour enhancers, thickeners and stabilisers, antioxidants, sweeteners, emulsifiers, food acids and preservatives. It is not always easy to spot food additives, as many are listed as E-numbers. To get the lowdown on what these different E-numbers represent, it is worth reading Maurice Hansen's excellent reference book *E for Additives* (Thorsons, 1984).

Processed, low-fat foods, such as cheese, yoghurts, mayonnaise and low-fat spreads should also be avoided as they are usually loaded with additives and some also contain hydrogenated vegetable oils.

Salt and salty foods can upset our blood glucose levels just as much as sugar, and salt is added to as many foods, so keep a lookout for it on product labels. These foods may not necessarily taste salty. For example, breakfast cereals often contain salt (listed as sodium). The majority of tinned foods, preserved meats, ready-made meals and snacks contain salt.

Beef and pork are the most difficult meats to digest and are likely to contain residues from the antibiotics and steroids that are routinely fed to the animals. These toxic residues make the meat even more difficult to digest and should be avoided. Try to eat organically reared beef and pork.

Smoked and burned foods are thought to contribute to stomach cancer if eaten in excess; however, there is no harm in treating yourself to a bit of smoked salmon every once in a while, or to the occasional barbecue.

Deep-fried foods are obviously going to be high in fat and therefore difficult to digest.

Drinks

You do not need to worry about drinking small amounts of tea
and coffee or combining them with other foods. However, if tea
and coffee are drunk close to meal-times they can interfere with
the absorption of certain nutrients. For example, if you drink
tea or coffee up to half an hour after a meal, it will destroy much
of the vitamin C gained from eating that meal. It is best to drink
beverages in moderation in between meals. Herb teas are a great
alternative to tea and coffee, which are both high in caffeine.
Fizzy drinks are best avoided as they can fill the stomach with air
and interfere with digestion.

MILK

Cow's milk should also be avoided as it is difficult to digest.
Many people are intolerant to cow's milk, which can exacerbate
colds, diarrhoea, catarrh and other conditions which involve an
excess of mucus. Unfortunately, most of us are led to believe
that cow's milk is our best source of calcium, but this simply is
not true; nuts, seeds, pulses and many vegetables are just as
good sources of this vital nutrient. Soya milk is often thought of
as a healthy alternative to cow's milk, but it is a processed food
which is also difficult to digest.

WATER

Drinking water is extremely good for us, as it helps to cleanse
our digestive system and replenishes our water supplies. We
should aim to drink about eight glasses of mineral water a day
in addition to other drinks. However, we should not drink
water with our meals as it dilutes the food and makes it pass too

quickly through the system without being fully digested. Leave a gap of half an hour before and after meals before you drink water. Avoid tap water as it contains several unhealthy chemicals including nitrates, chlorine and aluminium. Either drink pure mineral water or invest in a water filter which can sift out most of these undesirable substances. One of the best ways to cleanse your system morning and evening is to have a glass of hot water containing a slice of lemon. Lemon is a diuretic and it encourages the elimination of toxins.

ALCOHOL

Large amounts of alcohol should not be consumed as this will upset digestion, but to drink alcohol in moderation is fine for food combining. In fact, many studies have shown that a small glass of red wine a day is actually good for us, although this does not stretch to other forms of alcohol such as beer and spirits. Red wine contains antioxidant nutrients known as flavonoids. It is best to drink organic red wine, as most grapes are sprayed with pesticides and residues of these chemicals remain on the fruit during the vinification process. Drinking wine with your meal should not interfere with digestion as long as you drink in moderation, so don't worry about combining alcohol with foods.

JUICES

Fresh juices have the power to nourish, cleanse, protect, soothe and heal. They are nutritious and easy to digest and give us life energy in a naturally delicious drink. Most cartons of juice will contain additives and preservatives, so it is best to make your own juices with an electric juicer or blender. In addition, processed fruit juices turn acidic after lengthy exposure to the atmosphere. Juices are much more than just a drink, they are meals in themselves and one fresh juice will have more nutritional value than most of the processed meals available from supermarkets. It makes sense, then, to drink fresh juices every day. They are a delicious and refreshing way to reap all the nutritious benefits of fruit and vegetables and there are endless combinations.

In addition, fruit and vegetable juices help us to maintain and restore the correct acid–alkaline balance in the body. As we have seen, a typical Western diet, high in animal proteins, refined sugar and flour, chemical additives and drugs, causes acids to build up in the cell walls, which may eventually lead to complaints such as arthritis. Acid cells attract toxins which in turn make the cells more acidic. One of the main causes of fatigue is acidity of the blood and it's well known that cancer cells enjoy an acid environment. Fortunately, drinking a freshly made juice every day can rectify an unstable acid–alkaline balance as nearly all fruits and most vegetables are alkali-forming. To make your own juices, invest in a high-speed electric juicer, available from department stores at around £35. The best fruits and vegetables for boosting the digestive system are: beetroot, carrot, celery, cucumber, endive, grapefruit, lemon, papaya, pear, pineapple, radish, raspberry and watercress, so get juicing! For more information about the health benefits of juicing and great juice recipes see my *Quick Guide to Juicing* (Boxtree, 1994, £3.99).

6

Menu Planner
and Recipes

Breakfast

It is important to have some sustenance in the morning to
provide our bodies with the energy needed to keep us going
until lunch-time. If you have a proper breakfast, you are less
likely to have hunger pangs mid-morning and be tempted to
snack on a chocolate bar or piece of cake. As we have seen, it is
thought that between 4am and midday, our bodies are busy
eliminating the food we have eaten the day before. Therefore, in
order to boost our processes of elimination, it is best to eat
detoxifying fruit and vegetables for breakfast.

With its high water content, fruit is by far the easiest food to
digest and, because it passes quickly through the digestive
system, it does not consume the energy that the body needs in
order to carry out its processes of elimination. If you never feel
like eating in the morning, try having a freshly squeezed fruit or
vegetable juice instead. If a simple fruit juice is still too much for
you first thing in the morning, forsake your usual cup of tea or
coffee for a glass of hot water with a slice of lemon. Then, when
the hunger pangs hit you later on in the morning, try to eat fresh
fruit only and you can have as many pieces as you like. The best
fruits to eat are those with a high water content such as apples,
oranges, melon etc. If you have melon for breakfast, it is best to
eat it on its own as it has the highest water content of all fruits
and stays in the stomach for the shortest time. However, if you

find that these light fruits do not satisfy you, have a couple of bananas, which stay in your stomach longer than juicy fruits and are more filling. Always eat enough to feel satisfied, but never overeat! Another great breakfast is sliced banana mixed with some creamy, low-fat live yoghurt and a sprinkling of sesame seeds. It is best not to mix acid fruits with yoghurt, ie grapefruit, oranges, lemons and berries.

STARCH BREAKFASTS

The majority of boxed cereals are acid-forming, are made from wheat and contain added sugar and salt. These should be avoided, as food combining does not allow cereals to be mixed with milk. However, some people enjoy muesli with orange juice or water and lemon juice instead of milk and this is a healthy, acceptable combination.

Although it is best to have only fresh fruit in the morning, you can have the occasional starch breakfast, especially if you are not going to be able to eat again for many hours. Apart from muesli or porridge made with water (not milk) you can have toast with butter, jam, marmalade, honey, Marmite or maple syrup (but make sure that it is wholemeal toast!). If you do have a starch breakfast, then either your lunch or dinner should be wholly alkaline-forming as we are aiming for one alkaline meal, one starch meal and one protein meal every day.

BREAKFAST RECIPES
Wake-up Shake

This shake will boost your vitamin levels and give you extra energy at the start of the day. It tastes best chilled.

1 level tbsp sunflower seeds
1 level tbsp sesame seeds
2 apples – peeled and cored
1tsp crude blackstrap molasses
1 ripe banana (optional), peeled

Finely grind the seeds in a coffee mill or food processor. Liquidise the apples and bananas in the food processor and blend with the ground seeds and molasses. Serve immediately while still frothy.

Fruit Compote

This compote is the ideal fast-food breakfast as it is prepared the day before, can be kept in the fridge for at least a week and is ready to serve immediately.

> 350g (12oz) mixed dried fruit such as: apple rings, apricots, dates, figs, pears, raisins and sultanas
>
> 1/2 tsp allspice
>
> 1/2 tsp cinnamon
>
> 300ml (1/2 pint) water
>
> 50g (2oz) chopped almonds

Choose unsulphured fruit where possible. Soak the fruit and spices overnight in 300ml (1/2 pint) water. Serve with plain, live low-fat yoghurt and a sprinkling of chopped almonds.

Bircher Muesli

This recipe is based on the original muesli invented by Dr Bircher-Benner for patients at his famous natural health clinic in Switzerland. To save time in the mornings, the oats may be soaked overnight, leaving only the fruit and hazelnuts to be added at breakfast. Dr Bircher-Benner believed that the entire apple should be used – pips and all!

> Serves 2
>
> 4 tbsps rolled oats
>
> 2 tbsps low-fat, live yoghurt
>
> 6 tbsps cold water
>
> 225g (8oz) freshly grated (unpeeled) apple or 450g (1lb) seasonal soft fruits
>
> 2 tbsps chopped hazelnuts

Put the oats, yoghurt, water and lemon rind into a large bowl and stir until creamy. Leave in the fridge overnight if preferred. Add the fruit and serve sprinkled with chopped hazelnuts.

Hot Bulgar Breakfast

This delicious, nutritious hot cereal is a perfect winter warmer for cold, dark days. Serve plain or with additional milk or soya milk.
Serves 4

>   *1tbsp unrefined oil (eg virgin olive oil)*
>   *150g (5oz) bulgar wheat (cracked wheat)*
>   *100g (4oz) sesame seeds*
>   *100g (4oz) wheatgerm*
>   *600ml (1 pint) water*
>   *25g (1oz) dried apricots, finely chopped*
>   *25g (1oz) raisins or currants*
>   *25g (1oz) chopped hazelnuts or almonds*

Gently heat the oil in a large saucepan, add the bulgar wheat, sesame seeds and the wheatgerm, and lightly sauté until slightly browned. Add the water and stir in the dried fruits. Cover and simmer for about 25 minutes or until the bulgar is light and fluffy and the water has been absorbed. Add nuts to taste and serve immediately.

Snacks

It helps your digestive system if you leave a gap of four hours between meals, especially after a protein meal, so that each meal can be fully digested before your body has to get to work on the next load of food. However, if you are really hungry, you should not deprive your body of food. Snack on mainly neutral foods such as fruit, vegetables, seeds and nuts. If you fancy something sweet, dried apricots and currants are great to snack on, although their high sugar content makes them unsuitable for those who are on a diet.

If you are an incorrigible chocolate addict, try carob bars as a substitute. The long pods of the Mediterranean carob tree are used to make a sort of vegetable chocolate which is available as powder, 'chocolate' spread and in carob bars which are available from health-food shops and even some newsagents. Unlike chocolate, carob contains no caffeine and in its raw state is very low in calories and contains no fat. However, carob does not mix well with protein foods or those containing milk, so look out for these ingredients on the labels of carob products.

Unblanched almonds and raisins also make a tasty snack, but are high in calories.

Starch Recipes

If you fancy something light and low in calories, potatoes baked in their skins with a small dab of butter and a tasty salad is ideal. Alternatively you could have a salad sandwich. Those who are not trying to lose weight could have a creamy avocado sandwich.

Avocado and Alfalfa Sandwich Filling
A luxurious sandwich recipe which will fill you up with goodness.
Serves 1
1/2 avocado
1/2 spring onion, finely chopped
dash lemon juice
freshly ground black pepper
large handful alfalfa sprouts
2 thin slices wholemeal bread
Mash the avocado with the spring onion, lemon juice and black pepper and spread on a slice of bread. Sprinkle with alfalfa sprouts and top with the second slice of wholemeal bread.

Tahini and Cucumber Sandwich Filling

This is an instant and tasty snack. Tahini spread is made from crushed sesame seeds and is very high in calcium. It is available from good supermarkets and health-food shops.

Serves 1

1/2 tbsp of tahini spread
1 tsp chopped parsley
6 cucumber slices
2 thin slices wholemeal bread

Spread the tahini onto one of the slices of wholemeal bread. Sprinkle with the chopped parsley and place the cucumber and the other slice of bread on top. Serve with cherry tomatoes, radishes and spring onions.

Nut Butter

Nut butter and chopped celery make an unusual and tasty filling for sandwiches and baked potatoes in their jackets. But nut butter is far more versatile than just a spread – try dabbing a little over cooked carrots, or adding half a teaspoon to a salad dressing for extra flavour. (Cashew nuts have one of the lowest fat contents, but hazelnuts are fairly high in fat so use sparingly.)

450g (1lb) mixture of almonds, Brazil nuts, walnuts,
hazelnuts or peanuts
1/2 tsp sea salt
4 tbsps (60ml) apple juice

Roast the nuts in a medium oven for 10–15 minutes, stirring occasionally. Grind to a fine paste in a coffee mill or food processor with a sharp blade. Dry roast the salt in a pan over a low heat for 1–2 minutes and add to the nut paste. Stir in just enough apple juice to make a thick purée. Store in screw-top jars. If the natural oil in the nuts separates, simply stir it back in. You can also make this recipe using seeds. For seeds such as sesame or sunflower, dry roast in a pan over a low heat until the seeds crush easily when rubbed. Then proceed as before. If your butter ever develops mould in the jar, dispose of it immediately, as this can be lethal! Fortunately, this is very unusual.

Tabbouleh
Serves 6

> 175g (6oz) bulgar wheat (cracked wheat)
> 4 spring onions, trimmed and finely chopped
> 1 medium-sized cucumber, finely chopped
> 4tbsps freshly chopped parsley
> 1–2tbsps freshly chopped mint
> 1–2tbsps freshly chopped basil
> freshly squeezed juice of 1 lemon
> 60ml (4tbsps) cold-pressed olive or unrefined hazelnut oil

For the garnish

> 6 slivers red pepper or pimento
> 6 chopped black olives

Rinse the bulgar wheat thoroughly before soaking in cold water for at least an hour. Drain well. Add the finely chopped spring onions, cucumber and herbs to the lemon juice and oil and mix together well. Pour the mixture over the bulgar wheat and stir thoroughly. Serve garnished with red pepper or pimento and olives.

Buckwheat Bonanza
This buckwheat feast works well with the stronger flavours of wild mushrooms such as shiitake or oyster varieties.
Serves 2

> 50g (2oz) roasted buckwheat (kasha)
> 50g (2oz) buckwheat
> 450ml (3/4 pint) water
> 100g (4oz) artichoke hearts
> 1tbsp cold-pressed olive oil
> 100g (4oz) button or wild mushrooms, roughly chopped
> 4 spring onions, chopped
> 1tsp tamari sauce

freshly ground black pepper
25g (1oz) pecan nuts (optional)

Rinse the buckwheat in a sieve under a running tap. Bring the water to the boil, add the buckwheat, cover and simmer for 15 minutes or until soft. Meanwhile, if using fresh artichokes, trim and cook them in pure water or in a steamer. When soft, remove the leaves and trim away the toughened fibres to reveal the soft hearts. If using tinned artichoke hearts these will be precooked. Roughly chop the artichokes. In a large frying pan heat the oil and gently soften the mushrooms and spring onions. Drain the buckwheat and add to the pan with the chopped artichokes and herbs – stir well. Add the tamari sauce and freshly ground black pepper to season. Serve sprinkled with pecan nuts, if using.

Asparagus and Mushroom Risotto

To make this meal even more exotic, add a pinch of saffron to the cooking liquid to turn the rice yellow.

Serves 2

100g (4oz) brown rice (mixed if possible), well rinsed
475ml (16fl oz) water
1 large onion, peeled and finely chopped
few strands of saffron (optional)
100g (4oz) fresh asparagus, trimmed
100g (4oz) wild mushrooms, finely chopped
2tbsps chopped fresh parsley
freshly ground pepper
juice of 1/2 lemon

Gently heat a heavy-based saucepan on top of the stove, add the rice and stir with a wooden spatula for 1 minute until lightly toasted. Add the water, onion and saffron, if using. Bring to the boil, cover and simmer for 20 minutes. Meanwhile, chop the asparagus into short lengths, reserving the tips for the garnish. After 20 minutes add the lengths of asparagus and simmer for another 10–15 minutes until the rice is soft. In a separate pan, gently heat the olive oil and lightly sauté the asparagus tips. Remove from the pan and drain on kitchen paper. Stir the chopped mushrooms and parsley into the cooked rice mixture. Season with black pepper, stir in the lemon juice and serve garnished with the asparagus tips.

No-cook Rissoles

Serve these rissoles with one of the delicious salads listed in the neutral meals section (page 86–7).

Makes 8 small rissoles

   175g (6oz) mixed nuts (eg hazelnuts and almonds), ground
   100g (4oz) wholewheat bread crumbs
   1dsp finely chopped onion
   1tbsp chopped parsley
   1tsp low-salt yeast extract blended with 1tbsp water
   1dsp poppy or sesame seeds

Reserve about one-quarter of the nuts and breadcrumbs for coating, and mix all the remaining ingredients together. Form into small rissoles. Mix together the reserved nuts and breadcrumbs and use to coat the rissoles.

Barley and Vegetable Soup

This is a hearty, nourishing soup that satisfies the hungriest of stomachs and it works particularly well with root vegetables such as carrot, parsnip and swede.

Serves 4

   3tbsps cold-pressed olive oil
   2 onions, peeled and chopped
   450g (1lb) any colourful vegetable, chopped, diced or
      shredded
   75g (3oz) pot barley
   1/2tsp freshly grated root ginger
   1.2l (2 pints) vegetable stock
   freshly ground black pepper

In a large saucepan, heat the oil and lightly sauté the onions and the other vegetables of your choice. Stir in the pot barley, root ginger and stock, and season with the freshly ground black pepper. Cover and simmer over a low heat for 2 hours or until the barley is soft.

Three-seed Vegetable Risotto

I make plenty of this risotto as it keeps well in the fridge for 4–5 days. I then use it as a base for vegetable risotto or add it to soups and casseroles. It is also a favourite with my children and can be mixed with vegetable purées for a toddler's tea.

Serves 4–6

> 150g (6oz) long grain organic brown rice
> 75g (3oz) millet
> 50g (2oz) sunflower seeds (without shells)
> 4 large, ripe tomatoes, skinned and chopped
> 1tbsp olive oil
> 1 medium onion, finely diced
> 2 cloves garlic, crushed and chopped
> 1 low-salt vegetable stock cube (eg Friggs)
> 900ml (1½ pints) water
> 1tbsp low-salt yeast extract
> 1tbsp parsley, chopped

Rinse the grains and seeds in a sieve under cold running water and shake dry. Heat the oil in a frying pan and lightly sauté the onion and garlic until translucent. Add the mixed grains and stir for 2–3 minutes. Heat the water and dissolve the stock cube and yeast extract in it. Transfer to a large saucepan. Add the mixed grains and chopped tomatoes and bring to the boil. Reduce the heat, cover and simmer for 30–35 minutes or until the rice has cooked through. Sprinkle with chopped parsley and serve.

Pasta Pomodoro

This rich tomato sauce can be used for pasta, rice or fish. I always make twice the quantity as it keeps for up to a week in the fridge or in the freezer for three months. Passata (sieved tomatoes) is a good substitute for whole tomatoes and works well in this recipe. Cartons or jars of passata can be found in most supermarkets.

Serves 6–8
For the sauce:
    120ml (4fl oz) olive oil
    300g (10oz) onion, finely chopped
    4 cloves garlic, crushed
    1kg (2¹/₂lb) tomatoes, chopped or 1l (1¹/₂ pints) passata.
    1tbsp basil, chopped
    1tbsp oregano, chopped
Pasta:
    Allow 100g (4oz) dried wholemeal pasta per person

Heat the oil in a large saucepan or deep-sided frying pan. Add the onions, carrot and garlic. Stir frequently until the vegetables have softened. Add the chopped tomatoes or passata, cover the pan and simmer over a low heat for 20 minutes. Stir in the chopped herbs, partially cover and simmer for a further 10 minutes. Cook the pasta until al dente (slightly firm), drain and serve immediately with a helping of pomodoro sauce.

Brown Rice and Hazelnut Salad

This nutty flavoured salad is wonderful for a light summer supper.

Serves 4–6
    500g (10oz) brown rice, cooked
    75g (3oz) hazelnuts
    75g (3oz) currants
    50g (2oz) sunflower seeds
    4 spring onions, finely sliced

2tbsps parsley, chopped (reserve a few sprigs for garnishing)
1 dark lettuce, washed and trimmed
For the dressing:
2tbsps (30ml) sunflower oil
2tbsps (30ml) cider or white wine vinegar
2tsp (10ml) Dijon mustard
2 cloves garlic, crushed and chopped
1/2 tsp dried thyme
salt and black pepper

In a large bowl, toss the cooked brown rice with the hazelnuts, currants, sunflower seeds, spring onions and parsley. Mix the dressing ingredients together and pour over the rice salad. Stir well. Serve the salad in a lettuce-lined bowl and sprinkle with chopped parsley.

Cream of Celery Soup

This soup should ideally be served smooth, but it can also be prepared leaving out the puréeing stage.
Serves 4–6
1tbsp sesame oil
2 onions, peeled and finely chopped
10 stalks celery, chopped
40g (1 1/2 oz) oat flakes
1.25l (2 1/2 pints) water
1tsp freshly chopped thyme or dill

Heat the sesame oil in a saucepan and sauté the onions until transparent. Add the chopped celery and sauté for another few minutes. Stir in the oat flakes and gently cook for about 5 minutes until they are well coated with the sesame oil and moistened. Slowly stir in the water, cover and simmer over a low heat for 30–40 minutes. Purée the soup in a food processor until smooth. Serve sprinkled with the fresh herbs.

Cabbage Parcels

Serves 6
100g (4oz) millet
450ml (15fl oz) vegetable stock
1 savoy cabbage
1tbsp cold-pressed olive oil
2 red onions, peeled and chopped
4 spring onions, sliced into rings
8 stems of fresh coriander
2 cloves garlic, peeled and crushed
3 carrots, chopped
2 leeks, chopped
4 tomatoes, chopped
100g (4oz) okra, chopped
juice of 1 lime
freshly ground black pepper
2tbsps (30ml) water or stock

Preheat the oven to 180°C, 350°F (gas mark 4). Place the millet and stock in a saucepan, bring to the boil, cover and simmer for about 20 minutes or until the millet is soft. Separate the cabbage into whole leaves and blanch them in boiling water for 30 seconds. Set aside to drain on kitchen paper. Slice the stems off the coriander. Chop the leaves and set on one side.

Heat the oil and gently fry the onion, coriander stalk and garlic until the onion is transparent. Add the chopped carrots and leeks and continue to cook for another minute. Add the tomatoes, okra, the chopped coriander leaves and stir in the cooked millet. Add the lime juice and freshly ground black pepper to season.

Place a dessertspoonful of the millet mixture on a cabbage leaf and roll up, folding in the sides as you go. Repeat until all the cabbage leaves have been filled. Place in an ovenproof dish, spoon over the water or stock, cover and bake for 20 minutes.

Protein Meals

Lemon Chicken

Serves 4
1 free-range chicken
1 lemon
1 onion
1tbsp (15ml) olive oil
1 sprig of tarragon
25g (1oz) butter
freshly ground black pepper and sea salt to season

Preheat oven to 220°C, 425°F (gas mark 7). Peel the lemon and use the peel to stuff the chicken. Also add to this stuffing the onion, the sprig of tarragon, butter, some freshly ground black pepper and a little salt. Squeeze the juice from the lemon and use it to coat the outside of the chicken and add some salt and pepper. Place the chicken on parchment baking paper with a thin covering of olive oil. Bring up the sides of the baking paper to form a loose parcel and wrap this in an outer sheet of foil. Place in the oven for 20 minutes per lb plus 10–20 minutes extra. Halfway through cooking, remove the chicken from the oven and baste thoroughly. Open the top of the parcel for the last 10 minutes of cooking to allow the chicken to brown. Serve with steamed vegetables or salad.

Five-Vegetable Terrine

This multi-coloured terrine may be served hot or cold. For an attractive starter, slice and serve it in the centre of a plate of freshly squeezed tomato juice.

Serves 6–8
450g (1lb) carrots, diced
225g (8oz) celeriac, peeled and cubed
350g (12oz) fresh spinach
350g (12oz) broccoli, broken into florets

225g (8oz) leeks, white part only, sliced
freshly ground black pepper
juice of 1 orange
6 free-range eggs, size 3

Preheat the oven to 200°C, 400°F (gas mark 6). Cook the carrots and celeriac in boiling water in separate saucepans until tender. Cook the spinach in a little water for about 5–6 minutes. Blanch the broccoli and leeks in boiling water, separately, for 1–2 minutes. Drain all the vegetables well.

In a food processor, blend the leek and celeriac with a pinch of black pepper and two eggs until puréed to a coarse texture. Repeat, using the broccoli, spinach and two of the eggs. Finally, repeat the process with the carrot, adding the orange juice and two remaining eggs.

Line a 1kg (2lb) loaf tin with lightly oiled baking parchment paper. Spread the green spinach and broccoli mixture over the bottom and follow with a cream-coloured layer of leek and celeriac. Finally, top with a layer of carrot and orange purée. Place the loaf tin inside a large roasting tin filled with about 1cm (1/2 inch) of hot water. Bake for about 1 hour or until set. Turn out on a serving dish, allow to cool slightly then peel off the baking parchment before slicing the terrine.

Prawn Kebabs with Herb Dressing

Serves 2
For the Kebabs:
12 king prawns
8 button mushrooms
1 medium courgette, sliced
For the herb dressing:
4tbsps cold-pressed olive oil or unrefined sunflower oil
1 clove garlic, peeled and crushed
juice of one lemon
1 sprig each of basil, parsley and tarragon, finely chopped

Thread the prawns, button mushrooms and sliced courgette on to wooden or metal skewers and place in a shallow dish. Mix the ingredients for the herb dressing together thoroughly and pour over the threaded skewers. Cover and leave to marinate for 30 minutes, turning occasionally. Place under a medium heat grill and cook for about 3 minutes, basting and turning the kebabs as they cook.

Spicy Black Bean Soup

This is a hearty, warming soup that is especially welcome on cold, wet winter evenings. The chillies are excellent for unblocking the sinuses!

Serves 2

>   *150g (6oz) black-eyed beans, cooked*
>   *175ml (6fl oz) water or vegetable stock*
>   *1tbsp fresh tomato sauce or 1tbsp tomato purée*
>   *1 fresh red chilli, very finely chopped*
>   *1tsp olive oil (optional)*

Lightly fry the chilli in one tablespoon of olive oil and place in a saucepan with the cooked black-eyed beans, water or stock and tomato paste. Bring the soup to the boil, turn down the heat and leave to simmer uncovered for 10–15 minutes. Pour about two-thirds of the mixture from the saucepan into a blender and whizz for a few seconds. Return this to the remaining third in the saucepan, heat through and serve.

Green Bean and Bacon Salad

This colourful salad makes a tasty light lunch.

Serves 4

>   *450g (1lb) green beans, trimmed and sliced into 1½ inch*
>   *lengths*
>   *4 rashers lean unsmoked bacon*
>   *1 red pepper, deseeded and roughly chopped*
>   *1 small onion, finely chopped*

For the dressing:
> *150ml (5fl oz) natural, low-fat yoghurt*
> *1tbsp (15ml) olive oil*
> *1tbsp (15ml) lemon juice*
> *1tsp Dijon mustard*
> *2tbsp chopped chives*
> *1 clove garlic, crushed*
> *freshly ground black pepper*

Steam or microwave the beans in a small amount of water until tender, but still crisp. Trim the fatty rind off the bacon and grill. Cut into bite-sized pieces. Mix the beans, bacon and chopped raw onion and red pepper together. Stir all the dressing ingredients together and whisk. Pour the dressing over the salad and stir well.

Warm Goat's Cheese Salad

Goat's cheese is more easily digested than cheese made from cow's milk as its fat and protein molecules are smaller. This is because it is intended to feed a baby goat which, unlike a calf, is similar in size to a human baby.

> *Serves 4*
> *175g (6oz) goat's cheese*
> *1tbsp cold-pressed olive oil*
> *2tbsps Fine French dressing (see pages 87–8 for recipe)*
> *mixed salad leaves*
> *50g (2oz) pitted black olives*
> *50g (2oz) sunflower seeds*

For the dressing:
> *2tbsps (30ml) sunflower oil*
> *1tbsp (15ml) lemon juice*
> *1 clove garlic, crushed*
> *1tbsp fresh oregano, chopped*
> *salt and black pepper*

Preheat the grill or the oven to 180°C, 350°F (gas mark 4). Slice the goat's cheese into four thick slices. Brush a baking tray with the olive oil and place the cheese slices on it. Heat in the oven or under a medium grill until melted and lightly browned. Meanwhile, mix together the dressing ingredients, toss in the salad leaves and arrange on four small plates. Place one slice of goat's cheese in the centre. Sprinkle with sunflower seeds and olives and serve immediately.

Grilled Trout with Gazpacho Dressing

Serves 4

> 4 small trout
> 1 lemon
> freshly ground black pepper

For the dressing:

> 1/2 cucumber, roughly chopped
> 1 clove garlic, peeled and crushed
> 1/2 red pepper and 1/2 yellow pepper, deseeded and chopped
> 1 spring onion, sliced
> 1tbsp tomato purée
> 150ml (1/2 pint) olive oil
> 1tbsp (15ml) wine or cider vinegar
> 1tbsp fresh oregano, chopped
> salt and ground black pepper

For the garnish:

> 50g (2oz) watercress
> 1 lime, cut into quarters

Lay the trout out on a buttered piece of foil and cover with the juice of one lemon and some freshly ground black pepper. Put under a medium grill until the fish is cooked through, then arrange the trout on a shallow dish. To make the dressing place the cucumber, garlic, peppers and spring onion in a blender or food processor and whizz until finely chopped. Add the tomato purée, olive oil, vinegar and chopped oregano and process until smooth. Season with salt and pepper before pouring over the trout. Decorate with watercress and lime wedges.

Neutral Meals

Some of these neutral meals can be eaten on their own or they can be mixed with carbohydrate and protein foods.

Herbed Mushrooms

These mushrooms are delicious served alone as a starter or as a salad ingredient. They can also be drained and served warm as a vegetable side dish.

Serves 4–6

>   *450g (1lb) mushrooms*
>   *250ml (8fl oz) red wine vinegar*
>   *100g (4oz) onions, finely chopped*
>   *1tsp mixed spice, pickling spice or allspice*
>   *4 cloves*
>   *100g (4oz) red pepper, deseeded and sliced*
>   *120ml (4fl oz) sunflower oil*
>   *salt and freshly ground black pepper*

Lightly brush the mushrooms with a damp cloth to remove any earth. Blanch by plunging into boiling water for 20 seconds. Drain and allow to cool. Meanwhile, bring the vinegar to the boil in a non-aluminium pan. Add the chopped onions and seasonings. Cook for 2–3 minutes before adding the chopped red peppers, sunflower oil and salt and pepper. Cool the mixture, add the mushrooms and leave to marinate for 2–3 hours. Drain the oil and juices before serving. The mushrooms can be stored in a screw-top jar in the refrigerator for at least a fortnight.

Tapenade

This rich olive paste from Provence can be used to coat fish fillets, chicken breasts or cubes of tofu (all protein). Or simply serve it hot with a mixture of rices and green beans, or as an appetiser spread on small chunks of rye bread (carbohydrate).

Makes 175g (6oz)

> *100g (4oz) pitted black olives, chopped*
> *2tbsps capers, rinsed in milk to remove excess salt*
> *2 cloves garlic, peeled and crushed*
> *3tbsps extra virgin olive or hazelnut oil*
> *freshly ground black pepper*
> *chopped fresh oregano or basil or thyme to taste*

If using the tapenade to coat fish, chicken or tofu, preheat the oven to 180°C, 350°F (gas mark 4). Blend all the ingredients together in a food processor or pass them through a sieve to form a smooth paste. To coat the fish, chicken or tofu chunks, simply spread with the tapenade mixture and bake in the oven for 15–20 minutes.

VEGETABLE SOUPS

Vegetable soups are low in calories and rich in nutrients and they are especially quick and easy to make if you have a food processor or liquidiser. Make large amounts of soup and store in the freezer in portion sizes so that whenever you feel like some, you simply need to re-heat a portion.

The majority of vegetables are neutral and it is fine to add pasta or noodles to the recipes or enjoy some crusty bread and butter as an accompaniment. These additions would turn the soup into a carbohydrate meal. Alternatively, you may like to add some cream or grated cheese to your soup, in which case it would become a protein meal.

Vegetable Soup

This nourishing soup is quick and easy to make. It has exceptionally high levels of vitamin C and beta-carotene, and is a good nutritional booster.

Serves 4

> *125g (4oz) celery, chopped with its leaves*
> *125g (4oz) carrot, grated*
> *50g (2oz) raw spinach, finely chopped*
> *1l (1¹/₂ pints) water*
> *125ml (4fl oz) tomato juice*
> *1tsp honey*
> *¹/₂ tsp cayenne pepper*
> *1tbsp chopped chives*

Boil the water in a pan and add the chopped vegetables. Cover, turn down the heat and simmer for 20–30 minutes. Add the tomato juice, honey and cayenne pepper. Pour into the blender and liquidise until smooth. Serve with a sprinkling of chopped chives.

Onion Soup

Serves 2

> *2tbsps cold-pressed olive oil*
> *4 onions, peeled and finely sliced*
> *600ml (1 pint) vegetable stock, carrot juice or mixed vegetable juice*
> *dash of Worcestershire sauce*
> *pinch of freshly ground black pepper*
> *1 bay leaf*
> *2tbsps grated cheese (optional)*

Heat the oil in a large saucepan and fry the onions until transparent and soft. Add the stock or juice, the Worcestershire sauce, black pepper and bay leaf, cover the pan and simmer for at least 20 minutes to allow the full flavour to develop.

Carrot Soup

This soup is an amazingly good source of beta-carotene, but above all, it tastes delicious!

Serves 4

> *8 large carrots, scrubbed and sliced*
> *1.2l (2 pints) water*
> *1 low-salt vegetable stock cube (eg Friggs)*
> *1tbsp chopped coriander or parsley*
> *freshly ground black pepper, to season*
> *scant grating of nutmeg*
> *small carton plain low-fat yoghurt*
> *chopped chives to garnish*

Cook the carrots in the water with the vegetable stock cube. Add the chopped herbs and seasonings. Purée in a blender or a food processor until smooth. Serve in small bowls with a swirl of plain yoghurt and a sprinkling of chopped chives to garnish.

SENSATIONAL SALADS

Salads on their own are neutral and can be combined with either protein or carbohydrate foods. As there are so many different vegetables and herbs available there are unlimited ways of combining them to make delicious and nutritious salads. Here are a couple of suggestions:

Sunshine Salad

Serves 6

For the dressing:

> *150ml (½ pint) cold-pressed olive oil*
> *25ml (1fl oz) fresh lime juice*
> *2tsps French mustard*
> *freshly ground black pepper*

For the salad:

> *4 large carrots, scrubbed and grated*
> *225g (8oz) mixed salad leaves, such as spinach, radicchio,*

*frisée, oakleaf and batavia leaves, endive and lamb's
lettuce*
*50g (2oz) mixed herb leaves, such as chervil, basil and
roquette*
50g (2oz) sun-dried tomatoes, finely chopped
50g (2oz) hazelnuts, almonds or pecans, finely chopped

Mix together the dressing ingredients. Pour half the dressing over the grated carrots. Put the carrots in the centre of a large, flat serving platter. Arrange the mixed salad and herb leaves round the outside. Sprinkle with the chopped, sun-dried tomatoes and nuts. Pour on the remaining salad dressing and serve immediately.

Herb Salad

This tasty all-leaf salad makes a great accompaniment to pasta. Don't be tempted to make a more complicated dressing – let the herb flavours speak for themselves.

Serves 4
*300g (11oz) mixed salad leaves such as: spinach, radicchio,
frisée, chicory, rocket (arugula)*
*50g (2oz) mixed fresh herbs such as: chevril, basil, parsley,
coriander*
2tbsps (30ml) olive oil or walnut oil
1tsp (5ml) lemon juice

Simply toss all the ingredients together and serve.

DELICIOUS DRESSINGS

Dressings are the fastest way to liven up raw vegetables and salad combinations. The thicker ones based on yoghurt can also be used as dips for crudités.

Fine French Dressing

If stored tightly sealed in the fridge, this dressing will keep for up to a week.

Makes 300ml (1/2 pint)
    175ml (6fl oz) unrefined sunflower or safflower oil
    120ml (4fl oz) lemon juice
    freshly ground black pepper
    1/2 tsp mustard
    1/2 tsp freshly grated root ginger
    1–2 cloves garlic, peeled and crushed

Put all the ingredients in a screw-top jar, replace the lid and shake vigorously to mix well.

Cucumber Dressing

A delicious, refreshing dressing that also works well on sliced avocados.

Serves 2–4
    150g (5oz) cucumber
    150g (5oz) natural low-fat, live yoghurt
    1tbsp cider vinegar
    1 sprig of dill
    1/2 tsp dried dill seeds

Blend all the ingredients together in a food processor until the dressing is smooth and creamy.

Yoghurt and Chive Dressing (protein)

Serves 2–4
    150ml (1/2 pint) natural low-fat, live yoghurt
    1tbsp cold-pressed olive oil
    1tbsp lemon juice
    1tsp Dijon mustard
    2tbsps chopped chives
    1 clove garlic, peeled and crushed
    freshly ground black pepper

In a large bowl, mix all the ingredients together, adding black pepper to season, and stir vigorously. Alternatively, place ingredients in a large, screw-top jar, replace the lid and shake well.

Orange and Tamari Dressing

Tamari sauce is made from soya beans and is similar to soy sauce. Soya is a protein food but small amounts of tamari and soy sauce can be combined with carbohydrates without causing digestive problems. This particular dressing is ideal for raw spinach or salad leaves. It is also a useful dressing for those who dislike using vinegar.

Serves 2–4

> *150ml (¹/₂ pint) freshly squeezed orange juice*
> *1tsp grated orange peel*
> *2tbsps tamari sauce*
> *1tsp finely chopped fresh root ginger*
> *3tbsps cold-pressed olive oil*
> *1 clove garlic, peeled and crushed*

In a large bowl, mix all the ingredients together and stir well before using. Alternatively, put the ingredients into a large, screw-top jar, replace the lid and shake well.

Sumptuous Desserts and Sweet Snacks

Although the majority of puddings are not allowed on the food-combining diet, we all like to indulge ourselves occasionally. Here are a few recipes for healthy desserts. It is easier on your digestive system to eat these sweet snacks on their own or at least half an hour after a main meal.

Spiced Bananas

This recipe works well with pears too. Another way to make this dish is to bake the fruit in a preheated oven at 180°C, 350°F (gas mark 4) for 15 minutes to soften it, before pouring on the sauce and serving. Bake the bananas in their skins and they'll keep their colour better.

Serves 4

    4 large, ripe bananas
    50g (2oz) butter
    1tbsp clear honey
    2tsps allspice

Peel and slice the bananas and place in four individual serving bowls. In a small saucepan quickly melt the butter and stir in the honey and allspice. Pour over the bananas and serve immediately.

Courgette and Carrot Cake

This rich, dark cake tastes so delicious you won't believe it's so good for you! Butter is replaced with monounsaturated oil, which also makes the mixture fabulously moist. I add coarsely chopped walnut pieces for extra crunch, but if baking for small children these should be finely ground to avoid the risk of choking. I find that dipping the spoon into hot water before spooning out the molasses and honey enables these sticky sweeteners to slide off the spoon more easily.

Makes two 18cm (7inch) cakes

    2 free-range eggs, size 3
    2tbsps crude blackstrap molasses
    2tbsps clear honey
    150ml (1/2 pint) plus 1tbsp walnut, hazelnut or olive oil
    174g (6oz) buckwheat flour
    1tsp bicarbonate of soda
    50g (2oz) natural wheatgerm
    50g (2oz) chopped walnuts
    100g (4oz) carrots, scrubbed and grated
    100g (4oz) courgettes, washed and grated.
    4tbsps orange juice

Preheat the oven to 180°C, 350°F (gas mark 4). Lightly oil two sponge sandwich tins. In a large mixing bowl, beat the eggs together before adding the molasses and honey. Stir vigorously before pouring in 150ml (1/2 pint) oil. Fold in the buckwheat flour, bicarbonate of soda and wheatgerm, followed by the remaining ingredients. Pour into the baking tins and bake for 35–40 minutes, or until an inserted metal skewer comes out clean. Allow to cool before turning out and slicing into wedges. Store in a tightly sealed container in a cool place.

Strawberry Sorbet

This recipe can easily be adapted for use with other soft fruits such as raspberries or blueberries.

> *450g (1lb) fresh strawberries*
> *2tsps (10ml) clear honey (optional)*
> *juice of 1 large orange*

Blend the ingredients together in a food processor until smooth. Pour into a bowl or container and place in the freezer for an hour. Remove and allow the mixture to thaw a little, if necessary. Then beat well with a metal spoon to break up any ice crystals and return the sorbet to the freezer for at least 5 hours. Allow to soften at room temperature for half an hour before serving.

Glossary

Antioxidants – nutrients such as beta-carotene, vitamin C and vitamin E, which neutralise free radicals and so prevent cell damage.

Appropriation – the process of digesting food.

Assimilation – the process by which foods are absorbed and utilised by the body to create energy and repair cells.

Colonic irrigation – washing out the contents of the colon (the main part of the large intestine) with the use of water or other medication.

Diuretic – a substance that increases the flow of urine by promoting the excretion of salts and water via the kidneys.

Elimination – the removal of waste products from the body via the organs of elimination: bowels, liver, kidneys, skin, lungs and lymphatic drainage system.

Emulsifiers – food additives which mix two substances, such as oil and water, which do not normally mix.

Essential fatty acids – polyunsaturated fatty acids found in vegetable oils, nuts and seeds which are essential for the good health of all our cells.

Flatulence – discomfort caused by air trapped in the stomach.

Folic acid – a B vitamin which works in tandem with vitamin B12 to create new cells. It is an essential nutrient for pregnant women from the moment they conceive, as it can help prevent spina bifida in the first twelve weeks of pregnancy.

Free radicals – highly active and destructive oxidised particles which can cause cell damage.

Fructose – a fruit sugar which is now synthesised commercially for use as a sweetener. Unlike glucose, it does not stimulate insulin secretion and so does not contribute to hypoglycaemic attacks.

Gastric juice – the liquid secreted by the gastric glands in the stomach which contains hydrochloric acid to aid digestion.

Gluten – a mixture of proteins present in wheat that is a common cause of allergy in some people.

Hypoglycaemia – a deficiency of glucose in the bloodstream which causes muscular weakness and mental confusion. Commonly experienced by those on restricted diet and diabetics. If the condition is severe it can lead to hypoglycaemic coma. (Note the contrast with diabetic coma, which is caused by *hyperglycaemia*, or insulin deficiency.)

Useful Addesses

Organic Suppliers

Henry Doubleday Research Association
Ryton-on-Dunsmore, Coventry CV8 3LG
Tel: 01203 303517
This is the largest organisation of organic gardeners in the world and new members are welcome. Products and gardening books are available by mail order.

The Soil Association
86 Colston Street, Bristol BS1 5BB
Tel: 0117-929 0661
Their symbol is a consumer guarantee that food is high quality and genuinely organically grown, ie without the use of pesticides and fungicides. The Soil Association welcomes new members and can also advise on stockists of organically grown produce.

Health Associations

British Diabetic Association
10 Queen Anne Street, London W1M 0BD
Tel: 0171-323 1531

The British Digestive Foundation
3 St Andrews Place, London NW1 4LB
Tel: 0171-486 0341
The BDF funds research into all forms of digestive disease and offers practical guidelines to sufferers.

For details of your nearest colonic irrigation practitioner, send a SAE to the Colonic Irrigation Association, 31 Eaton Hall, Eaton College Road, London NW3 2DE. Tel: 0171-483 1595

Index